EaseLife Protocols

Ease the pain and discomfort of life, with EaseLife protocols in natural ways and without any drugs.

by

Dr. Sujala Ainapure

Shilpa Abhyankar

Book Title:
EaseLife Protocols

Author:
Dr. Sujala Ainapure
Email: ainapuresujala@gmail.com

Co-Author:
Shilpa Abhyankar
Email: shilpa@enrichlife.org

First Edition: 1.4.2020
Second Edition: 15.1.2024

Notice

Neither the Publisher nor the Editor assumes any responsibility for any loss or injury and/or damage to persons or property arising out of or related to any use of the material contained in this book. It is the responsibility of the treating practitioner, relying on independent expertise and knowledge of the patient, to determine the best treatment and method of application for the patient.
The Publisher

Printed in Mumbai, India

About the Author

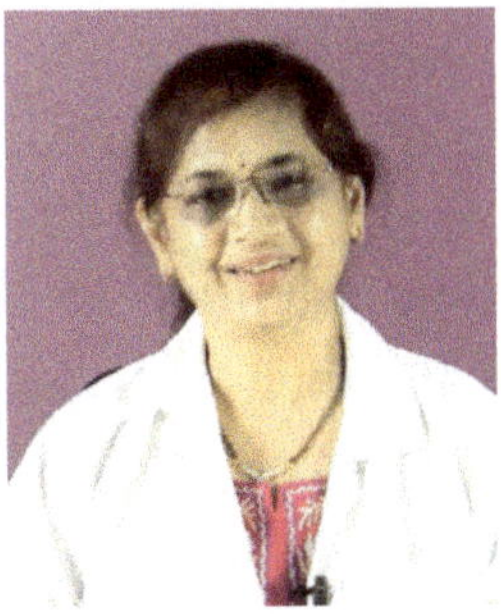

Dr. Sujala Ainapure is an eminent allopathic MD doctor with 35+ years of experience. She has a broad-minded approach and keen passion to help her patients. This prompts her to explore several alternate and natural ways to heal ailments and promote health. She is very generous and eager to share her knowledge for helping others. This book is an example of the same.

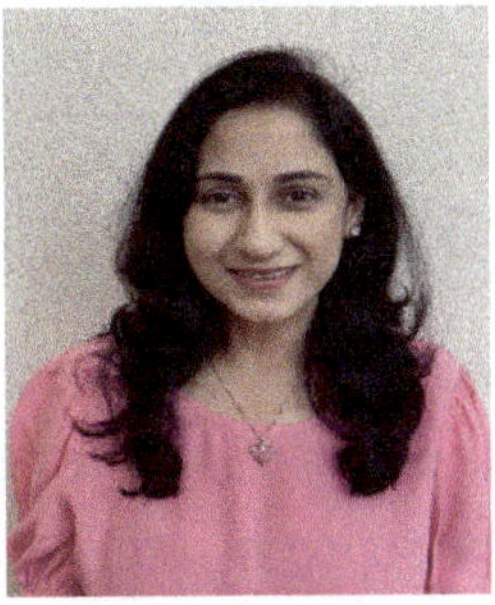

Shilpa Abhyankar has been a holistic health and life coach for the last 15 years. She is certified in several natural therapies. Her passion is to guide, treat and empower people in their journey from "Suffering to Smile". With this goal, she has conducted many workshops to teach people about these therapies in USA and India. She founded the practice of EnrichLife which combines techniques of Sujok Therapy, Acupressure, Yoga-Meditation, Hypnotherapy, and Ayurvedic Nutrition.

Disclaimer

The intention to share this knowledge is pure and giving. Having said that, individuals differ in terms of energy and preferences. Therefore, please use these protocols as you see appropriate and per your discretion. Diagnosis is of prime importance. Please consult your physician for proper diagnosis and use of this protocol. Also apply your own judgement prior to use of any method. No one holds any liability towards the results.

Dedicated to my father,

Mr. M. P. Khedkar, whose encouragement and interest in my work, has inspired me to develop these protocols and share them with all of you.

Foreword

EaseLife Protocols is the product of Dr. Sujala Ainapure's genius. Early in her career she realized that Allopathy, in which she is trained with a postgraduate degree, does not have answers to many sufferings. Even when it has remedies, there are a lot of difficulties associated with the treatment. Unlike most medicos, who accept the limitations of allopathic treatment, she decided to research and learn different techniques that can help her patients.

She first trained herself in acupuncture followed by acupressure and Sujok. She enthusiastically learned the science and encouraged patients to try alternative treatment along with mainstream medicine as required. Her integrated approach to healing was very effective. I am a witness to her efforts in selflessly propagating the treatments for the benefit of ailing people.

She has treated multitudes of patients in the hospital where both of us work, with results that are rewarding and at times magical. She has provided relief from years of suffering and prevented the need for several surgeries. I have personally tested some of the protocols developed by her and experienced their effectiveness.

She has never taken any credit for her work, which she says is the wish of some higher power. Her only purpose of publishing the book is to disseminate the knowledge acquired by years of experience.

I know that every element of the book is true, and the book will change the perspective from treatment to healing. Doctors and others alike will hugely benefit from the knowledge.

Best,

Dr. Nisha Shah
MD Pediatrics

Testimonials

The book "EaseLife Protocols" by Dr. Sujala Ainapure is very unique.

In this book, she has explained her innovative application for treating pain and discomfort in the simplest way. This can be very effectively used as a first-line treatment for common ailments with faster relief and ease in the symptoms. In many cases, instant relief can be observed.

The technique is explained very systematically in this book. It can be easily mastered and practiced. Simplicity and quick results are the key to this innovative application.

This treatment modality will be very useful for the masses and especially in our country where the ratio of health professionals to people is very low. In such a scenario, "EaseLife Protocols" would filter out many cases.

I am an acupuncture practitioner. At times, I also find it inconvenient to call patients for repeat sessions of acupuncture in simple pain cases. But now with "EaseLife Protocols", I have experienced that the patient gets instant relief of around 40 to 60% and further relief is obtained in a relatively short period of time without frequent additional visits.

I hope this book will help to guide many therapists to give relief to their patients.

Shripad Chodankar
Registered Acupuncture Practitioner & Teacher
(Ph.D.) in Acupuncture
Founder of Panacea Point Clinic

Preface

Welcome! This eBook shares protocols for treating several health issues using Acupressure, Acupuncture and Sujok techniques. The protocols were identified during my practice in treating many patients in the long tenure. I was highly impressed and sometimes astonished to see magical results from these protocols.

As an allopathic doctor, I have seen patients mainly treated through drugs, diet, physiotherapy, occupational therapy, and surgery. However, there are limitations to this approach. All the intricacies of body-mind and health are still not fully understood by Medical Science. As a doctor, I was eager to help all my ailing patients coming with hope. This prompted me to explore other alternate therapies.

Acupuncture was the first amongst them. In Acupuncture/Acupressure, several points on the body including the ear, can be used for healing. I started using Acupuncture in chronic cases, which had failed to respond to any other allopathic treatments for a long time. Among these were a five-year-old child who had developed foot drop due to nerve palsy and had not responded to expert physiotherapy for 6 months, two cases of frozen shoulder suffering for more than 9 months and a 52-year-old Osteoarthritis knee patient suffering from pain. All of these showed more than 75% improvement in just 3 weeks of acupuncture therapy. Success in these cases truly opened my mind to alternative therapies.

I came across Sujok Therapy, developed by South Korean Scientist, Professor Park Jae Wu. According to him, Nature clearly indicates its Purpose, its Love and tries to help human beings stay healthy. In Sujok therapy, our entire body is mapped on hands/feet using different correspondence systems. Initially, it was hard to scientifically understand and accept all of these different systems. However, I was surprised when they all worked effectively in treating different cases. I fell in love with Sujok therapy. It uses simple tools such as seeds, magnets, color and pressure on hand and feet to treat symptoms in natural ways.

The success of these therapies further opened my outlook towards healing methods. These methods are simple, effective, with low cost and hardly any side effects. It highly encouraged me to have an integrated approach for treatment. I continued to identify simple and natural means which can decrease the patient's visits to doctors. That is how I discovered protocols to treat several conditions.

I am extremely thankful to my dedicated Acupuncture teachers, Dr. T.C. Tolia and Dr. P. B. Lohiya. They are both allopathic doctors, practicing and teaching acupuncture. My deepest gratitude to the Sujok originator, Prof. Park Jae Wu for discovering, researching and sharing this amazing therapy to the world. I am also grateful to my patients who put their faith in me and contributed to the development of these protocols. Special thanks to my dear friend Mrs. Namratha Akkireddy for helping me compile the data and write this book. I am thankful to my sister Mrs. Pradnya Kanade for doing illustrations in this book and my daughter-in-law, Dr. Anjali

Raghunath who has done the cover pages and helped in editing this book. My sister, Mrs. Shilpa Abhyankar was also inspired to learn Acupuncture and Sujok. She has been practicing for the last 10 years and has partnered with me to complete this book. Mrs. Ashlesha Kelkar contributed to the electronic formatting of the book. My father, Mr. M.P. Khedkar has been a great source of inspiration to me. He encouraged me to continue learning and developing new protocols. Seeing the benefits, he chose to learn Acupuncture at the age of 75 yrs. and Sujok at the age of 82 yrs.

My hope is that these simple, relatively easy, and reasonably practical protocols can benefit the greater population. As a healer, the intention of the therapist plays a big role in all energy work. All the best and happy healing.

Regards,

Dr. Sujala Ainapure
MBBS, DCH, MD (Pediatrics),
Certified Acupuncturist and Certified Sujok Practitioner

Index

Basic Concepts

Treatment Therapy

Prior knowledge of Acupressure/Acupuncture and Sujok is required in understanding the protocols. Please use the reference diagrams for implementing the treatment location and method.

In Acupressure/Acupuncture, energy / 'chi' is flowing through certain meridian pathways in the body and when these pathways are blocked, disease manifests. Specific points on these meridians are identified for unblocking the stagnated energy to promote healing. Treatment is given utilizing these points on the body.

Any change or blocks in the energy channels can be brought about by external influences such as injury, infection, climate changes and lifestyle stresses (faulty eating and sleeping habits, extreme/ less physical activity, and wrong postures). Internal influences can be brought about by vibrations created by negative emotions. This may generate wrong electrical signals that flow to every cell in the body, which can result in malfunctioning of the cells and organs and may even influence the mental state of the person.

As the larger channels of energy lie close to the surface of the organism, they can be manipulated using pressure, needles, tubes, seeds, and other methods.

On restoring the correct flow in the larger channels, the smaller channels at cellular level are also restored, improving the health condition.

In Sujok therapy, our entire body is mapped on hands/feet using different correspondence systems. Therefore, our hands/feet can be used as remote controls to treat any part of the body using these systems.

The meridians of the body can be represented on our hands and feet. This system is called Byol meridians. Through this system, all the acupoints can now be identified on hands/feet for treatment.

In addition, the human ear is also a correspondence system of the entire body and can be used for healing as per the Auricular system.

System References

1. Sujok Standard Correspondence (Standard CR*): Single palm
2. Sujok Insect Correspondence (Insect CR): Single finger
3. Sujok Animal Correspondence (Animal CR): Single thumb
4. Sujok Mini Correspondence (Mini CR): Upper phalanx of the finger
5. Byol Meridians - These are Acupressure meridians on hand correspondence
6. Ear Acupressure (Auricular) - in this system, the body is mapped on the Ear

*** Correspondence is denoted as 'CR' in this book.**

Reference Diagrams

1. Sujok Standard Correspondence (Standard CR*): Single palm

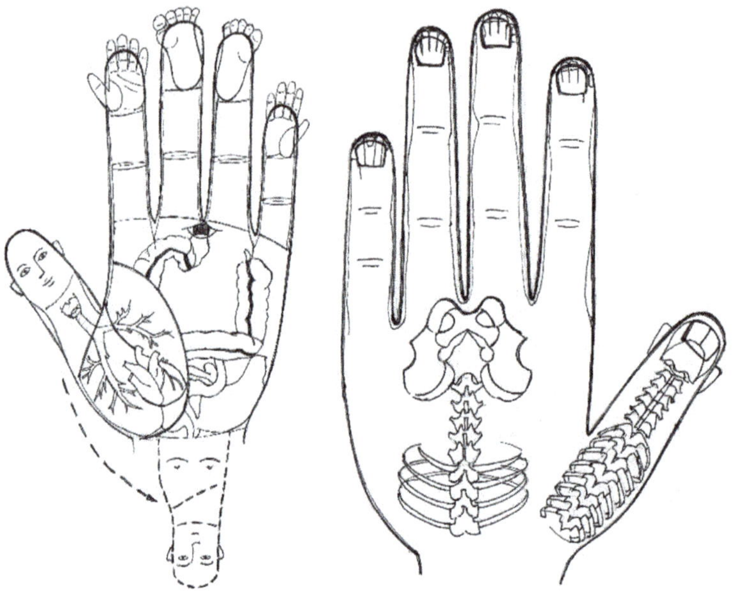

Front of the Left Hand
(Ventral side)

Back of the Left Hand
(Dorsal side)

Fig 1: Sujok Standard Correspondence (Standard CR)

2. Sujok Insect Correspondence (Insect CR): Single finger

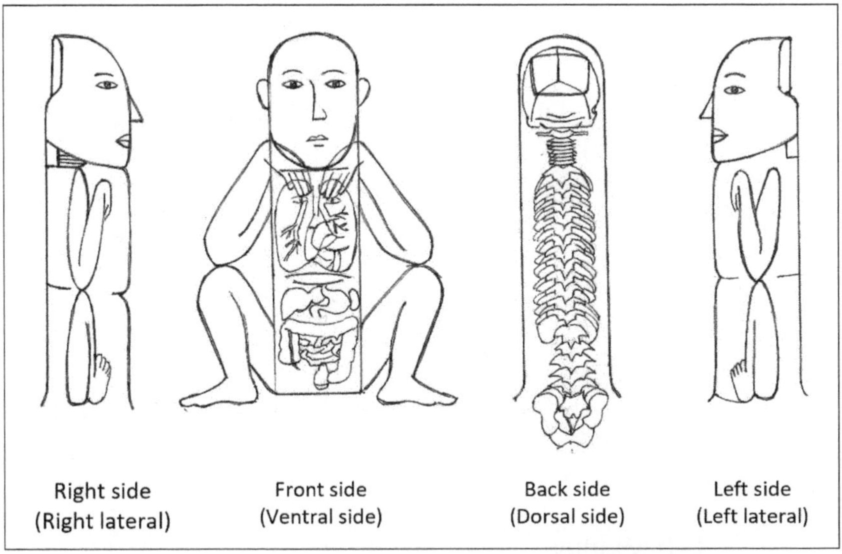

Fig 2: Sujok Insect Correspondence (Insect CR)

3. Sujok Animal Correspondence (Animal CR): Thumb or any other finger

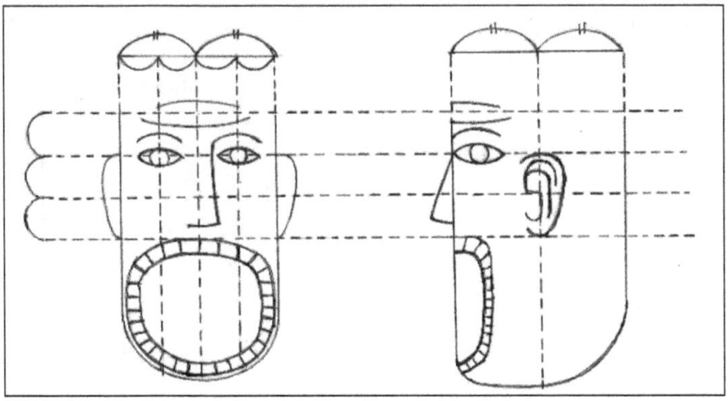

Fig 3: Sujok Animal Correspondence

4. Sujok Mini Correspondence (Mini CR): Upper phalanx of the finger

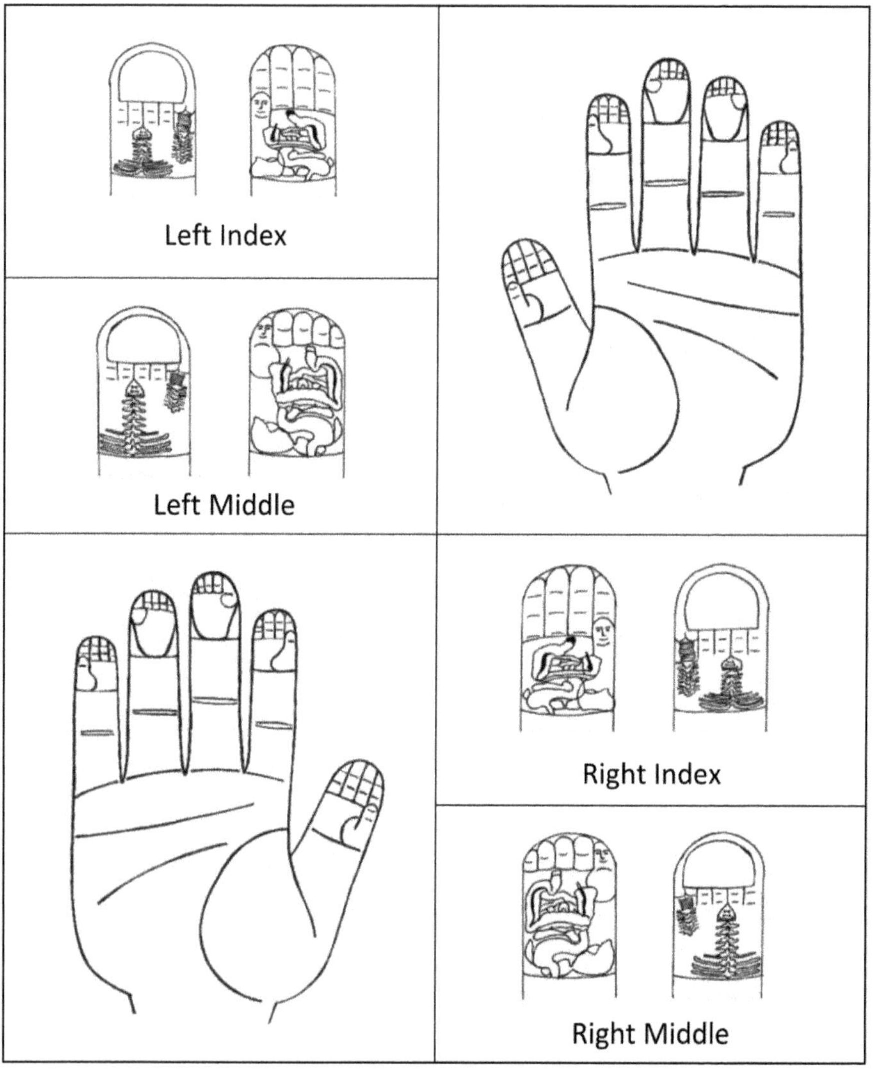

Fig 4: Sujok Mini Correspondence (Mini CR)

5. Byol Meridians - These are Acupressure meridians on hand correspondence

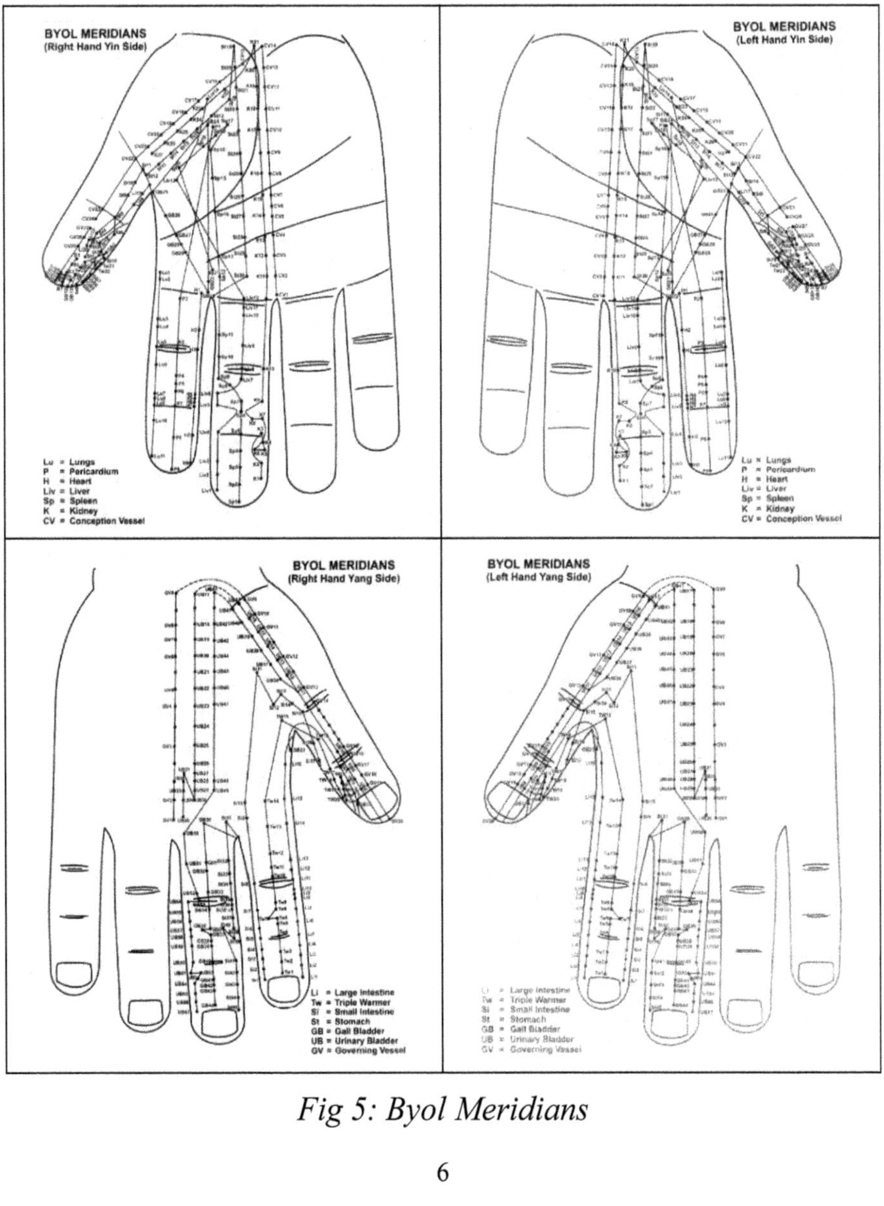

Fig 5: Byol Meridians

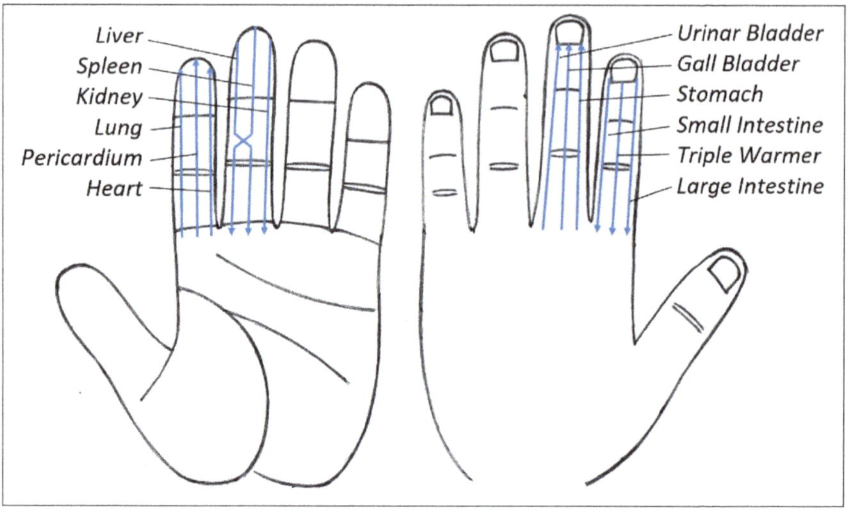

Fig 6: Byol Meridian lines on fingers

6. Ear Acupressure (Auricular) - in this system, the body is mapped on the Ear

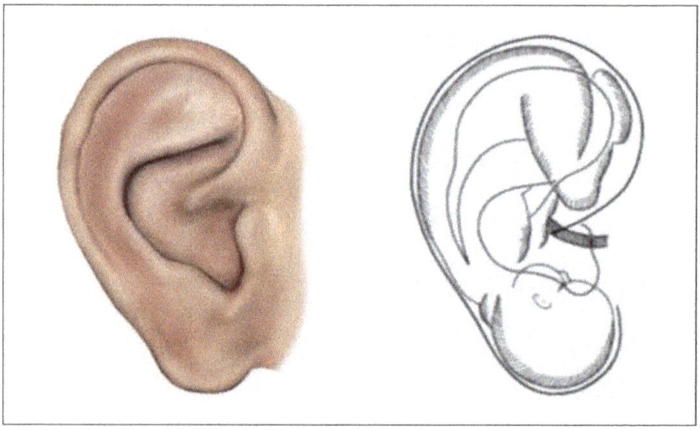

Fig 7: The body mapped on the Ear

*** Correspondence is denoted as 'CR' in this book.**

Treatment Modes

There are 6 different modes of treatment used in this series. A particular health issue can use any combination of these modes. Please choose the sequence of treatment methods based on the preference of the therapist and receptivity of the patient.

The method which we found more successful in my practice is mentioned at the end of introduction of each protocol. Table in Annexure 1 of this book gives an idea about the time taken for recovery. This table states the data about recovery period of patients undergoing therapies (either individually or in combination) mentioned in EaseLife protocols.

This data was collected retrospectively over a period of 3 years.

1. Tube - Nontoxic plastic hollow tube is applied in a particular direction of a correspondence system for the given condition.
2. Acupoints - Acupressure with Jimmy and seeds are used at relevant acupoints on Byol meridian correspondence.
3. Ear - Ear needle or seeds are used on the ear correspondence (Auricular therapy).
4. Bleeding - A sterile blood-letting instrument like lancet or needle is used to bleed few drops at an appropriate correspondence.
5. Wheat - Wheat seeds are applied in a particular direction, using a correspondence system that is appropriate for the given condition.

The reference diagrams described earlier clarify the correspondence system we are using and identify the specific location of treatment.

Before proceeding with the therapies described ahead, please watch the video titled 'Essentials of EaseLife Protocols' from the YouTube channel named 'EaseLife Protocols'. You can copy the link below and paste it on to your browser.

Video link:

https://www.youtube.com/watch?v=YgX8eoaoTpU

Channel link:

https://www.youtube.com/channel/UCbRAjFndufbDiZnYk9yxreg/videos

Patient testimonials can be viewed on the above-mentioned YouTube channel to give an idea about the results of these therapies.

Basic Material Used for Treatment

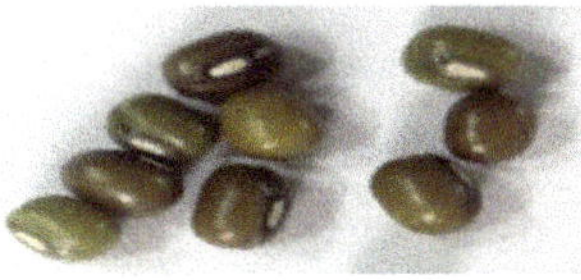

Moong Seeds

Non-Toxic Hollow Plastic Flexible Tube Pieces

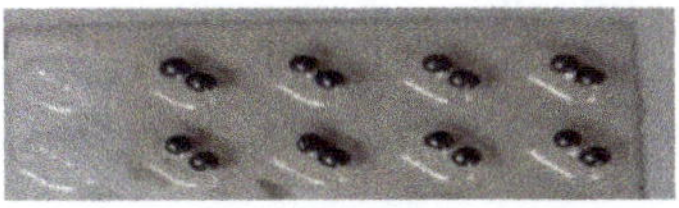

Ear Seeds

Ear Needles

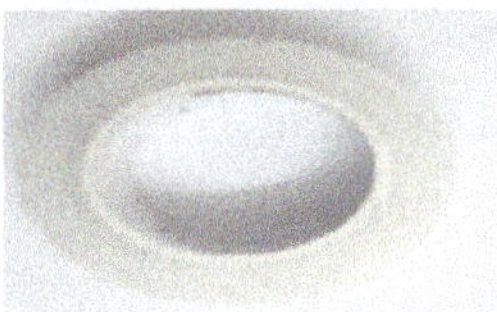

Non-Toxic Medical Adhesive Tape

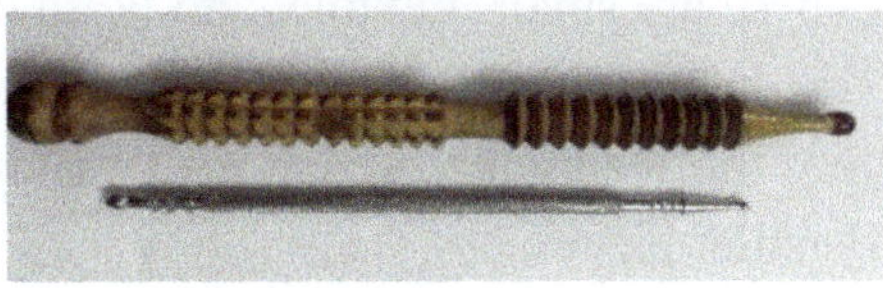

Jimmy

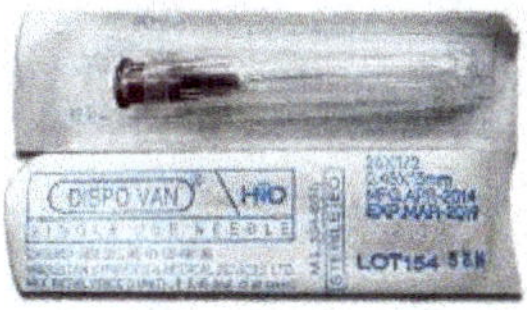

#26 Disposable Needle

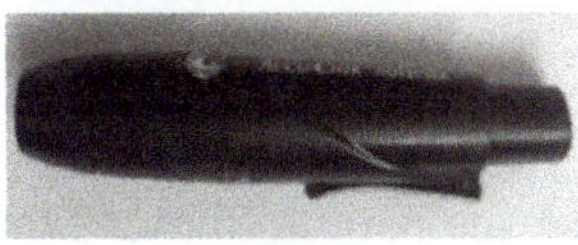

Bloodletting Instrument

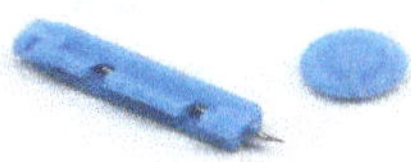

Blood Lancet

Bloodletting Instruments

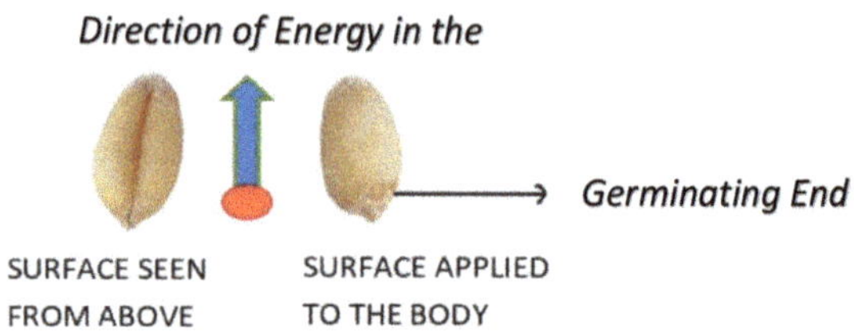

Wheat Seeds

Fig 8: Material used for the Treatment

Mode of Treatment - Tube

- Nontoxic plastic tubes are to be used to channelize energy. These are small, flexible, and hollow tubes, between ½ inch to 1½ inch in length. The hollow diameter can be about 1-2mm. For this technique, we cut the IV (intravenous) infusion set into smaller pieces.
- Sujok maps the affected part of the body on either hand or feet using various correspondences.
- Roll Jimmy on the Area of affected Correspondence.
- Apply the tube with an adhesive tape in the defined direction at CR as per the protocol.
- After 2-3 minutes, ask the patient to move the affected part and reassess the pain. If there is some definite relief after applying the tube (>10%), then retain the tube in that position for

36 - 48 hours. Application of the tube for a longer duration can damage the skin.

- Moving or shifting of the tube from its place can decrease or even nullify the effect. If needed, secure the tube position with an additional non-toxic adhesive tape like Band-aid. It should neither be too tight to cause excessive pressure/pain nor too loose to displace the tube from its position.
- Removing the tube before the specified time can decrease or nullify the effect.
- Once removed, it must be reapplied for 8-10 hours at the exact same location every day, till the problem completely disappears.
- **Kindly note that even when the pain disappears completely, the associated tissues are undergoing repair. They should not be unduly stressed and ideally given rest for 3-7 days depending on the extent and type of injury.**

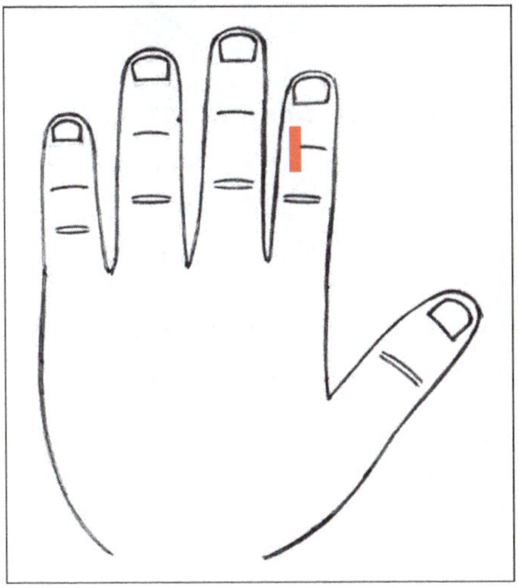

Fig 9: Tube Treatment

Mode of Treatment - Acupoints

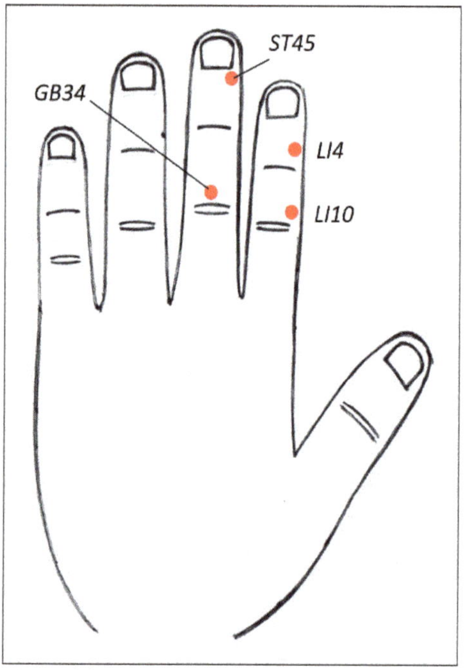

Fig 10: Acupoints Treatment

- This mode uses Sujok correspondence and Byol meridians.
- ACPJ - uses acupressure with the tool, Jimmy.
- ACPS - uses acupressure with seeds.
- Stimulate the labeled points by giving moderate pressure with jimmy on the Byol meridians for 3 - 5 seconds.
- For example: GB34, ST45, LI4, LI10.

- If the pain has not totally disappeared after applying firm pressure on these points with jimmy, then apply moong seeds on the same points with the help of non-toxic adhesive tape. Moong seeds are neutral seeds. We have used them in most protocols and are denoted by 'ACPS'.
- On the first day, ask the patient to press these seeds every 2 hourly (30 times in a minute) till bedtime.
- Remove the seeds in the morning after pressing them again the same way.
- Thereafter, apply for only 8 hours a day, till complete recovery. Press immediately after application and then at the end of 8 hours before removal. It is easier to apply seeds before bedtime and remove them in the morning.
- Each day, use fresh seeds.
- Continue for 2-20 days as required. For convenience in remembering, you can mark the points using henna (Mehendi) whenever needed.
- After 20 days give rest for 1week and then seeds can be applied again if required.
- **Please note that the Acupoints are mostly tender. They should be pressed well to get the effect, but in accordance with the patient's tolerance.**

Mode of Treatment - Bleeding

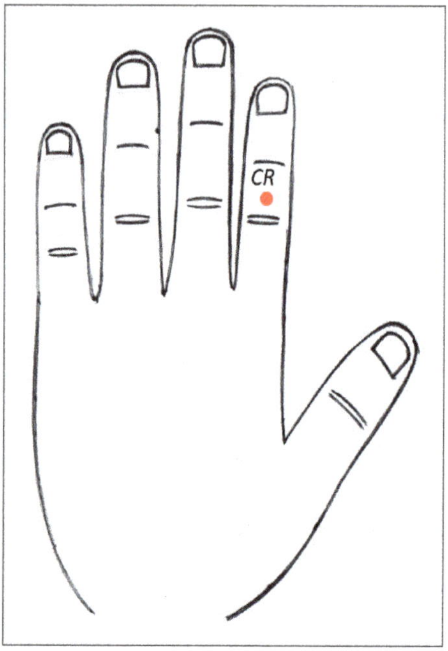

Fig 11: Bleeding Treatment

Bleeding from a point help to drain stagnated energy at greater speed. Even if the point bleed just 1 to 2 drops or does not bleed after prick, it is helpful in draining stagnated energy.

- Find out the highly tender correspondence point (CR) with jimmy.
- Gently massage the point.
- Clean the area with alcohol (clinical spirit).

- Prick the point with a sterile blood-letting instrument and bleed 8 to 12 drops of blood with aseptic precautions. Therapists should wear sterile gloves as a precaution.
- Ensure that bleeding has stopped after the procedure.
- **Bleeding should be followed by application of tube on the same point, to give further relief.**

Mode of Treatment - Ear Seeds

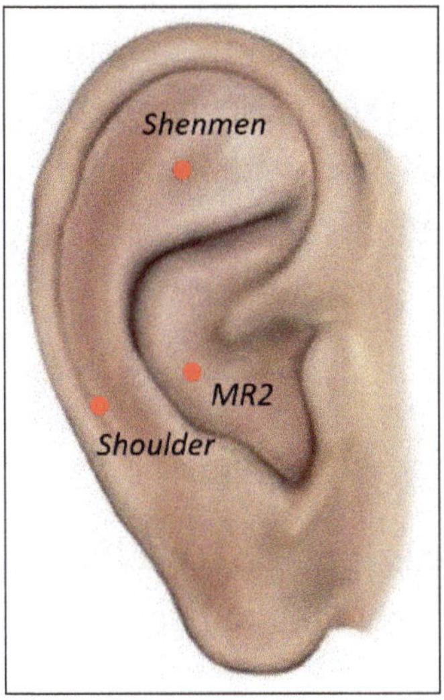

Fig 12: Ear Seed Treatment

- Check the ear points for tenderness with the help of Jimmy or a point finder. For example, points like - Shoulder, Shenmen, MR2 (muscle relaxing point).

- Clean the ear with clinical spirit to maintain asepsis and to improve the adhesion of tape to skin.
- Ear seeds / ear press needles are applied at these points. These are to be retained for up to 2-4 weeks. We have used vaccaria seeds (single or dual) for this method of treatment.
- Pressing the ear seeds by the patient is beneficial. It can be done twice a day (20- 30 times each) if the point is not very tender.
- The patient should be given proper instructions regarding care to be taken. Do advise not to rub or touch the seed often and protect it from water.
- Sometimes, the ear press needle may move from its position and cause severe pain. In such a scenario, the patient can remove the ear press needle on his own. Ear seeds are preferred over ear press needles due to this reason.

Mode of Treatment - Wheat Seeds

- Apply wheat seeds on the specified points such that the germinating end, where the red dot is shown in the figure, must be placed on the skin.
- After applying the wheat, ask the patient to wait for 20 minutes. Usually there is some relief in the symptoms during this period.

- Wheat seeds should be kept for 4-12 hours during the first 2 days.
- The patient is required to confirm improvement and then only continue the treatment. Use fresh wheat seeds daily.
- If there is aggravation of the symptom or discomfort, then the wheat seeds should be removed immediately, and some other method should be tried.
- If there is no exaggeration, then keep wheat for 4 hours before discarding this mode of treatment.
- Continue this type of treatment for 2-20 days as required.
- After 20 days, give a resting period of 1 week and then the seeds can be reapplied.
- In acute cases, treatment should be discontinued once complete relief is obtained.
- In chronic cases, treatment is tapered over time before discontinuing, for example reduce the time and frequency per week.

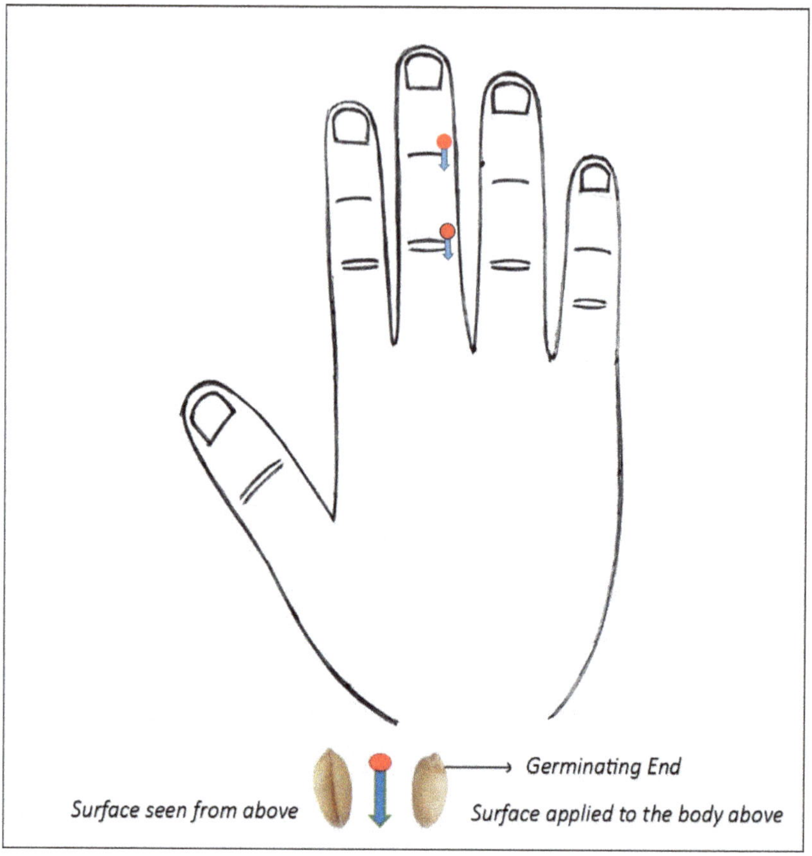

Fig 13: Wheat Seed Treatment - UB Meridian sedation

Special Instructions

1. Explain the complete procedure to the patient before starting treatment.
2. It is good practice to have the patient lie down or sit comfortably during the therapy.
3. Ensure that the patient is not on an empty stomach. On an empty stomach, there is a chance that the patient may feel dizzy during the treatment.
4. In rare cases, the patient may feel dizzy due to sudden shift in energy or as a reaction to pain. This particularly happens when he has an empty stomach or is weak or scared. In such a scenario, make the patient lie down immediately and ask him to take deep and slow breaths and give him an energy drink.
5. Pregnant women and very old patients should be treated with caution.
6. Explain the basic care to be taken by the patient and any follow-up if required.
7. The patient needs to duly follow the instructions for the success of the treatment.
8. For any muscular pain, particularly recurrent type, please rule out any Vitamin D deficiency disorder. In Vitamin D deficiency, spasm can be recurrent and severe.

9. **EaseLife protocols are simple ways of addressing common problems, but it is not a panacea. If the condition of the patient does not improve, then please see an expert in the field for accurate diagnosis and treatment.**

10. Before proceeding with the therapies, please watch the video titled 'Essentials of EaseLife Protocols' from the YouTube channel named 'EaseLife Protocols'. You can copy the link below and paste it in your browser. Also watch testimonials to get an idea about the effect of protocol.

    Video link:

    https://www.youtube.com/watch?v=YgX8eoaoTpU

11. **The therapist should imagine the affected part on the given correspondence while performing the therapy, as given in the respective protocols (shown in the figure).**

Protocols

1. Acute Neck Sprain

Introduction

A neck sprain is quite a common condition and can cause significant discomfort.

Here person commonly presents acutely with pain, causing significant restriction of movements of neck in one or more directions.

It usually occurs because of improper movement while exercising, lifting weight, or adopting a wrong posture for a prolonged time (while sleeping/ reading/ watching TV/ working on computer) causing strain to the ligaments or muscles.

For this condition, we found acupoints stimulated by Jimmy followed by moong seed application most effective.

Please refer to the Mode of Treatment details and watch the accompanying video from the 'Basic Concepts Chapter' before proceeding to the specific protocol described ahead.

Acute Neck Sprain - Tube

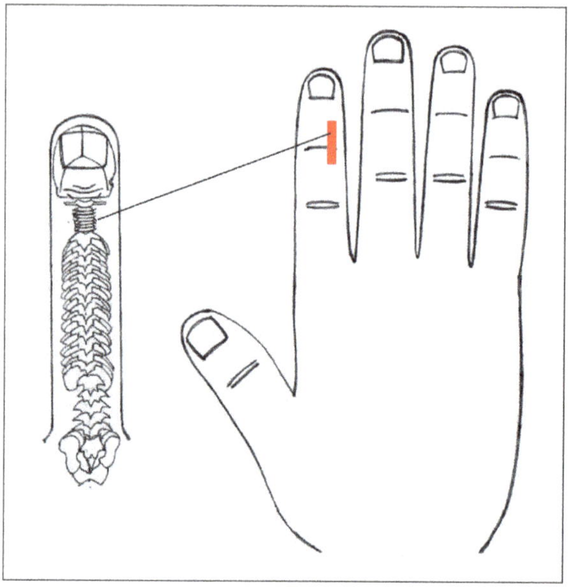

Fig 1.1: Treatment for Acute Right-sided Neck Sprain using Insect CR on Right hand

- Roll Jimmy over the Area of the affected neck region in Insect CR of index or any other finger.
- Identify the tender CR point and the direction of maximum tenderness based on the distribution of pain (vertical/horizontal/slanting).
- Apply a hollow plastic tube in the identified direction at the CR point (usually vertical) to get relief.
- Ask the patient to move the affected part and reassess the pain after 2-3 minutes.

- If there is some noticeable relief after applying tube (>10%), then retain the tube in that position for 36 - 48 hours. Its position must be well secured by Band-aid like tape (it should neither be too tight to cause excessive pressure nor too loose to cause displacement of the tube).
- Moving the tube from its place can decrease or even nullify the effect.
- Once removed, it must be reapplied for 8-10 hours, at the same location, every day till the problem completely disappears.

Acute Neck Sprain - Acupoints

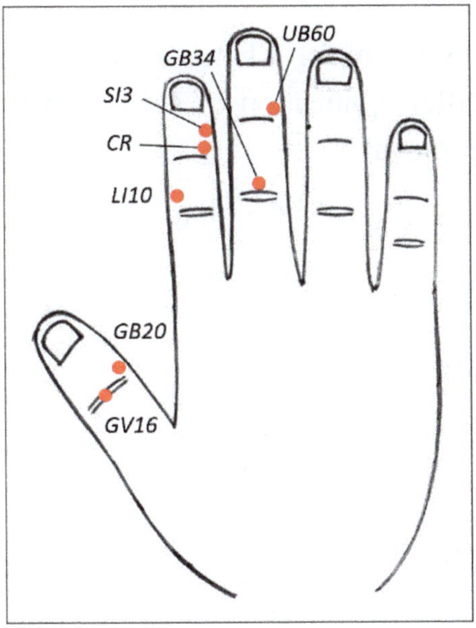

Fig 1.2: Acupoint Treatment for Acute Right-sided Neck Sprain using Byol Meridian

- Stimulate and apply pressure on the following points of Byol meridians using a jimmy. Choose the same hand as that of the site of the neck pain. For neck pain in the center, any hand is ok.

  These points are: GB20, SI3, LI10, GB34, UB60, GV16, CR (Ah Shi point).

- If the pain has not fully disappeared after stimulation with jimmy, then apply moong seeds on the same points with the germinating part (opening) touching the skin with an adhesive tape.
- On the first day, ask the patient to press these seeds 2 hourly (30 times in a minute).
- Thereafter, apply only for 8 hours a day till recovery, pressing immediately after application of seeds and at the end of 6-8 hours before removal.
- Every day use fresh seeds. Continue for 1-15 days as required.

Acute Neck Sprain - Ear Seeds

- Check the following points for tenderness with the help of jimmy or point finder.
- Neck, Shenmen, Muscle Relaxant point2 (MR2)
- Ear seeds are applied at these points after cleaning the ear.
- Ear needles are applied with aseptic precautions.

- These are retained for 2-3 weeks.
- Explain to the patient the essential safety instructions to be followed while using this therapy.

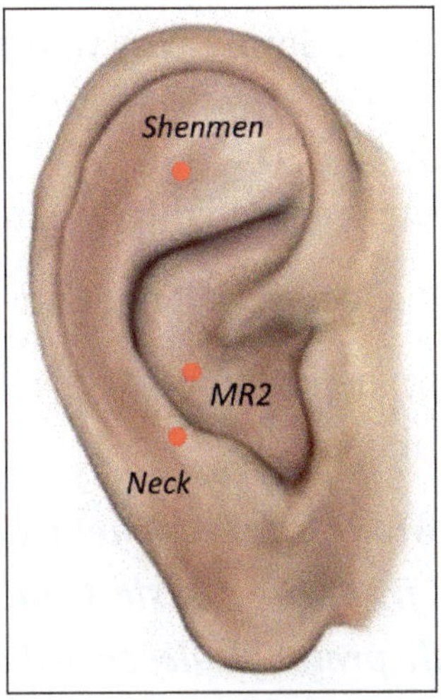

Fig.: Ear Seed Treatment for Acute Right-sided Neck Sprain using Ear Seeds

2. Acute Neck Pain

Introduction

This is a distressing condition usually due to

- Sudden jerk in the neck during play or otherwise.
- Wrong sleeping posture.
- Working on computers or studying for prolonged time.
- Acute pain in chronic cervical spondylitis.

In this condition, we found acupoints with seeds and tube application most useful.

Please refer to the Mode of Treatment details and watch the accompanying video from the 'Basic Concepts Chapter' before proceeding for specific protocols described ahead.

Acute Neck Pain - Tube

- Roll Jimmy on Area of the affected neck region on Insect CR on index or any other finger.
- Identify the tender CR point and apply a hollow plastic tube with an adhesive tape in the effective direction (usually vertical at the CR point).
- Review the pain and ask the patient to move the affected part after 2-3 minutes of tube placement.

- If there is some definite relief after applying the tube (>10%), then retain the tube in that position for 36 - 48 hours, its position must be well secured by an additional Band-aid-like tape. (It should neither be too tight to cause extra pressure nor too loose to move the tube from its place.)
- Displacement of the tube can decrease or even nullify the effect.
- Once removed it has to be reapplied for 8-10 hours every day, at the exact same location, until the problem completely disappears.

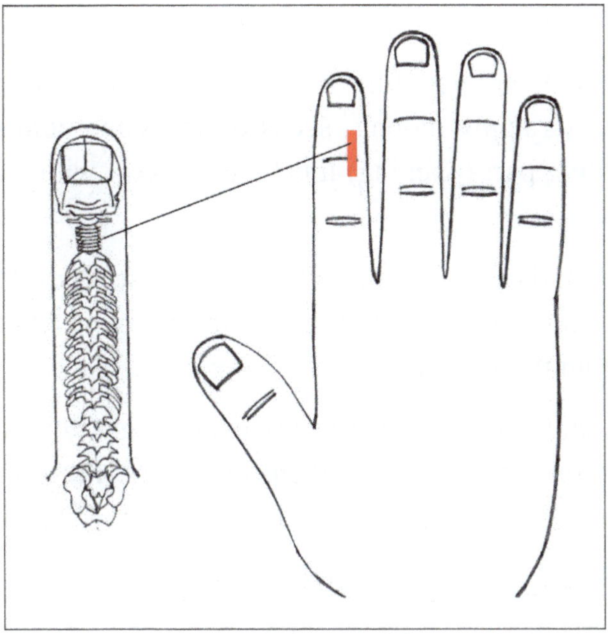

Fig 2.1: Treatment for Acute Right-sided Neck Pain using Insect CR on Right Hand

Acute Neck Pain - Acupoint

- Stimulate the following points lying on the Byol meridians by giving pressure with a jimmy. Choose the same hand as that of the site of neck pain (Left hand for left sided neck pain and right hand for right sided neck pain. For neck pain in the center, any hand is ok).
- The points are: GB34, GB20, SI3, UB60, LI10, GV16 and CR (Insect CR on Index finger). For chronic pain add GV4, GV14, UB11, UB23, K3, K7 For location of these points refer to fig. 13.2 on page 91.
- If the pain has not fully disappeared after stimulation with jimmy, then apply moong seeds on the same points with the germinating part (opening) touching the skin with an adhesive tape.
- On the first day, ask the patient to press these seeds 2 hourly for 30 times/minute. Remove them in the morning after pressing them again the same way.
- Subsequently, apply fresh seeds every night. Press them 30 times in one minute. Keep them overnight. Press them again after waking up in the morning and then remove the seeds.
- Continue for 2-20 days as required.
- After 20 days, give a break for 1 week and then the seeds can be applied again.

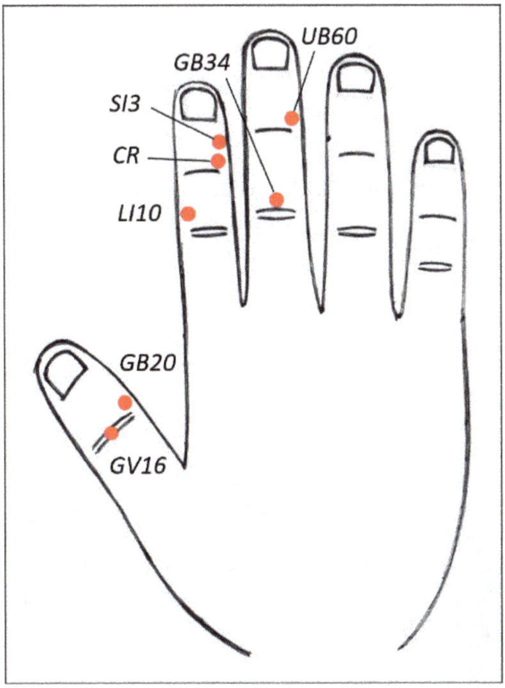

Fig 2.2: Acupoint Treatment for Acute Right-sided Neck Pain using Byol Meridian

Acute Neck Pain - Bleeding

- Find out the most tender CR point with Jimmy.
- Gently massage the point.
- Clean the area with clinical spirit.
- Prick the point with a sterile blood-letting instrument and then bleed 8 to 12 drops of blood under aseptic precautions.

- This method is especially useful when there is a history of an injury caused by sudden jerking of the neck. (For example, while playing basketball).
- Apply a hollow plastic tube over the point that is bled. Follow tube protocol for further relief.

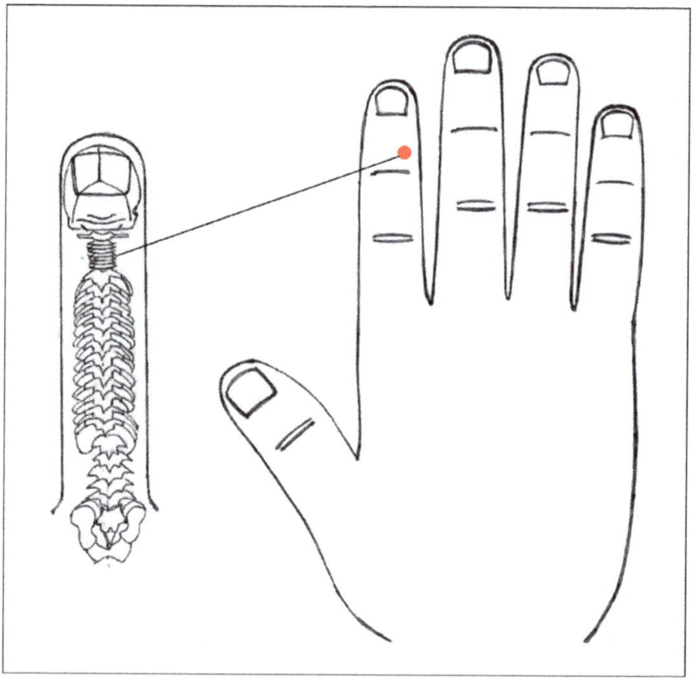

Fig 2.3: Bleeding Treatment for Acute Right-sided Neck Pain using Insect CR

Acute Neck Pain - Ear Seeds

- Check the following ear points for tenderness with the help of a jimmy or point finder.
- The points are Neck, Shenmen, MuscleRelaxant2 (MR2).
- Ear seeds are applied at these points after cleaning the ear.
- These are retained for 2-3 weeks.
- The patient should be given instructions on the basic care to be taken.

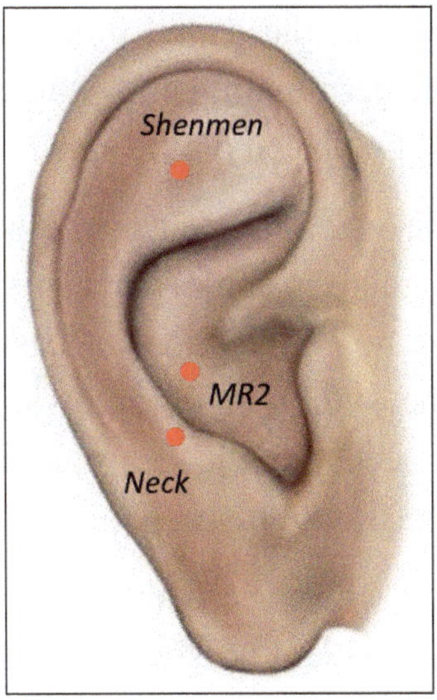

Fig 2.4: Ear Seeds Treatment for Acute Right-sided Neck Pain

Acute Neck Pain – Wheat Seeds

- Neck Pain along the meridian, SI or UB is common and can be treated by sedating the particular meridian using wheat therapy.
- If neck pain is associated with pain radiating to the arm (along SI meridian), then check for tenderness on the Jing well point SI1. If tender, apply wheat seeds as shown in the figure.
- If neck pain is associated with upper back pain, then check for tenderness on the point, UB67 (Jing well point of the UB meridian). If tender, apply wheat seeds on this meridian as shown in the figure.
- Apply wheat seeds on the stated points (as per the meridian used), such that the germinating end, where the red dot is shown in the figure, must be placed on the skin.
- After applying the wheat seed, ask the patient to wait for 20 minutes. Usually, there is some relief in symptoms during this period. If there is no relief, then at least there should be no aggravation of the symptom or untoward symptom. In such cases, the wheat seeds should be removed immediately, and some other method should be tried.
- For the first 2 days, wheat seeds should be kept for 8-12 hours during the day. The patient is asked to confirm improvement before continuing this treatment.
- Every day use fresh wheat seeds.

- Continue for 2-20 days as required. The duration of the treatment should be tapered when more than 70% pain relief is experienced.
- Treatment should be discontinued once complete relief is obtained.

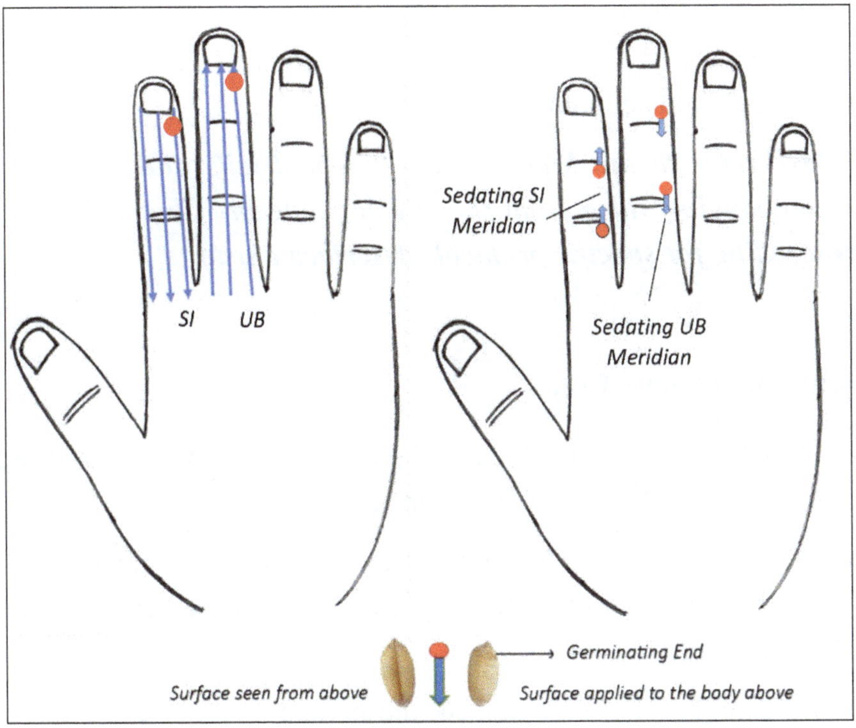

Fig 2.5: Wheat Seed Treatment for Acute Right-sided Neck Pain

3. Acute Back Pain

Introduction

Acute back pain without any known cause or injury is usually due to muscular spasm or ligament strain. Patients complain of acute pain in the upper / mid / lower back or Paraspinal region.

For this condition, acupoint GV26 stimulated strongly by Jimmy for 4 -5 seconds was found to be beneficial followed by tube application and acupoints.

Please refer to the Mode of Treatment details and watch the accompanying video from the 'Basic Concepts Chapter' before proceeding for specific protocols described ahead.

Acute Back Pain – Tube

- Roll Jimmy over the Area of the affected back region in Insect CR of the index or any other finger.
- Identify the tender CR point and apply a hollow plastic tube with adhesive tape in the effective direction (usually vertical at the CR point).
- Re-examine the pain and ask the patient to move the affected part after 2-3 minutes of tube placement.

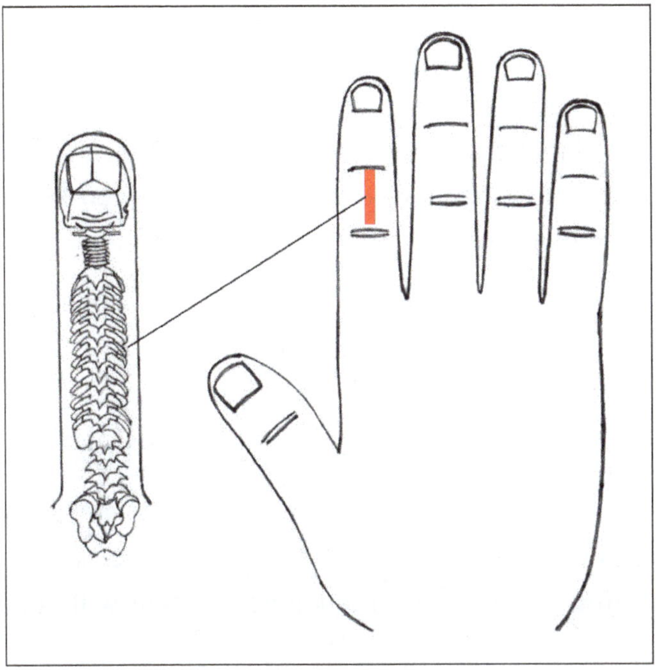

Fig 3.1: Tube Treatment for Acute Back pain in thorax region using Insect CR

- If there is some definite relief after applying the tube (>10%), then retain the tube in that position for 36 – 48 hours, its position must be well secured by an additional Band-Aid-like. (It should neither be too tight to cause extra pressure nor too loose to move the tube from its place.)
- Displacement of the tube can decrease or even nullify the effect.
- Once removed, it must be reapplied for 8-10 hours every day, at the exact same location, until the problem entirely disappears.

Acute Back Pain - Acupoints

- Stimulate the following points by giving pressure with jimmy on the Byol meridians. Choose the same side hand as that of the pain. Alternate moong seed application between left and right hand if the pain is in the center.
- **First try stimulating the point, GV26 for 4-5 seconds with good pressure. This single point can bring relief in most cases (watch testimonial of Acute Back pain).**
- If not, try the following points: GB34, SI3, UB62, CR.
- If the pain has not fully disappeared after stimulation with jimmy, then apply moong seeds on the same points with the germinating part (opening) touching the skin with an adhesive tape.
- On the first day, ask the patient to press these seeds 2 hourly for 30 times/minute. Remove them in the morning after pressing them again the same way.
- Subsequently, apply fresh seeds every night. Press them 30 times in one minute. Keep them overnight. Press them again after waking up in the morning and then remove the seeds.
- Continue for 2-20 days as required.
- After 20 days, give a break for 1week and then the seeds can be applied again.

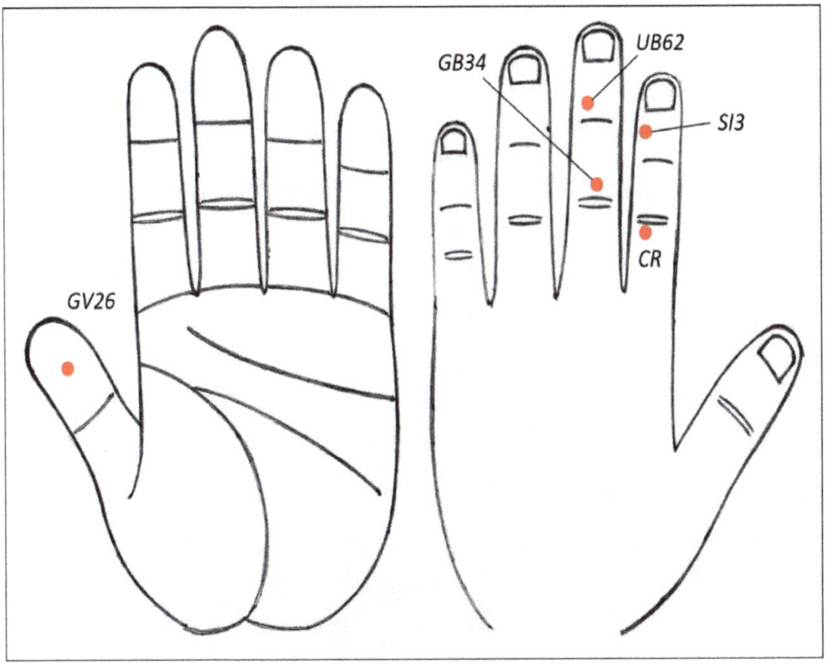

Fig 3.2: Acupoint Treatment for Acute Back pain in thorax region using Byol Meridian

Acute Back Pain - Ear Seeds

- Check the following ear points for tenderness with the help of jimmy or point finder.
- The points are: Shenmen, Muscle Relaxant1, Muscle Relaxant2, CR.
- Ear seeds are applied at these points after cleaning the ear.

- These are retained for 2-3 weeks.
- The patient should be given instructions on the essential care to be taken.

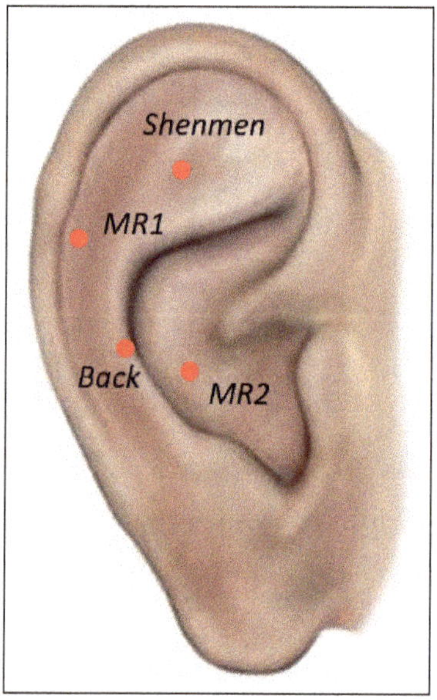

Fig 3.3: Treatment for Acute Back pain in thorax region using Ear Seeds

4. Acute Shoulder Pain

Introduction

The patient presents with shoulder pain of varying intensity. The cause is generally due to unaccustomed exercise, sleeping in odd ways, and prolonged use of the arm without proper rest.

In this condition, tube application and acupoints with seeds has been effective.

Please refer to the Mode of Treatment details and watch the accompanying video from the 'Basic Concepts Chapter' before proceeding with the specific protocol described ahead.

Acute Shoulder Pain – Tube

- Roll Jimmy over the Area of the affected shoulder region in Insect CR of index or any other finger.
- Identify the tender CR point and apply a hollow plastic tube with an adhesive tape in the effective direction (usually vertical at the CR point).
- The CR point which is tender can be either on the dorsal or lateral aspect of the finger.
- After 2-3 minutes, ask the patient to move the affected part and review the pain.

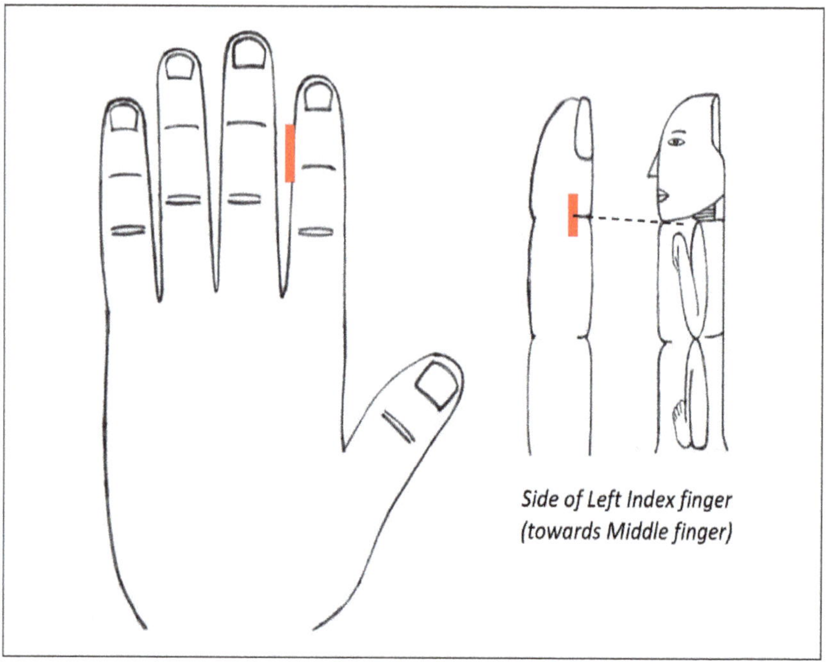

Fig 4.1: Treatment for Acute Left Shoulder Pain using Insect CR on Left Hand

- If there is some definite relief after applying tube (>10%), then retain the tube in that position for 36 - 48 hours. Its position must be well secured by an additional Band-aid like tape (it should neither be too tight to cause pressure nor loose so that the tube can move from its place).
- Moving the tube from its place can decrease or even nullify the effect.
- Once removed it must be reapplied for 8-10 hours every day, at the same location, until the problem fully disappears.

Acute Shoulder Pain - Acupoints

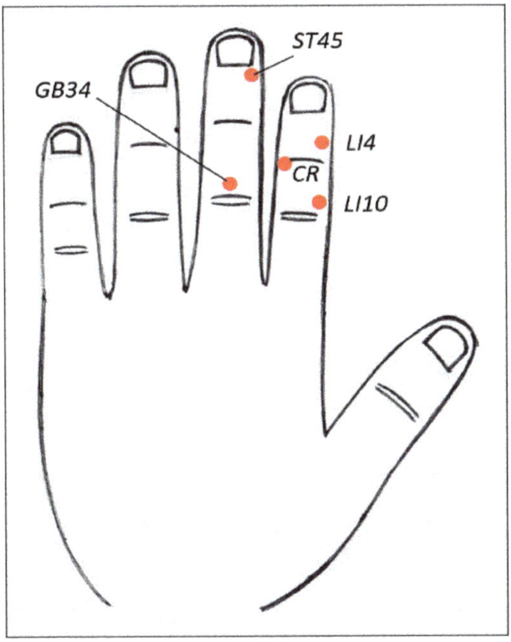

Fig 4.2: Treatment for Acute Left Shoulder Pain using Byol Meridian on Left Hand

- Stimulate the following points by creating pressure with jimmy on the Byol meridians. Choose the same side hand as that of the pain.
- The points are: GB34, ST45, LI4, Li10, CR.
- If the pain has not fully disappeared after stimulation with jimmy, then apply moong seeds on the same points with the germinating part (opening) touching the skin with an adhesive tape.

- On the first day, ask the patient to press these seeds 2 hourly for 30 times/minute till bedtime. Remove them in the morning after pressing them again the same way.
- Afterwards, apply fresh seeds every night. Press them 30 times in one minute. Keep them overnight. Press them again after waking up in the morning and then remove the seeds.
- Alternate between left and right hand if the pain is in the center. Continue for 2-20 days as required.
- After 20 days, give rest for 1 week and then the seeds can be applied again.

Acute Shoulder Pain – Bleeding

- Find out the highly tender point in Insect CR using Jimmy.
- The CR point which is tender can be either on the dorsal or lateral aspect of the finger.
- Gently massage the point.
- Clean the area with alcohol (clinical spirit).
- Prick the point with a sterile blood-letting instrument like lancet/needle and bleed 8 to 12 drops of blood with aseptic precautions.
- Apply a hollow plastic tube over the point that is bled. Follow tube protocol for further relief.

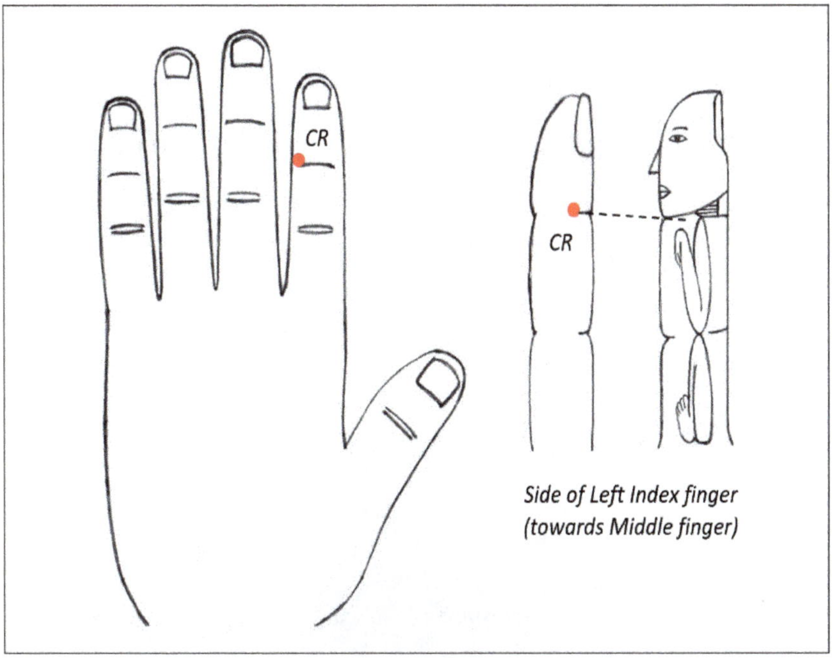

Fig 4.3: Treatment for Acute Left Shoulder Pain using Insect CR on Left Hand

Acute Shoulder Pain - Ear Seeds

- Check the following ear points for tenderness with the help of a jimmy or point finder.
- The points are Shoulder, Shenmen, Muscle relaxing point2 (MR2).
- Ear seeds are applied at these points after cleaning the ear.

- These are retained for 2-3 weeks.
- The patient should be given instructions on care to be taken.

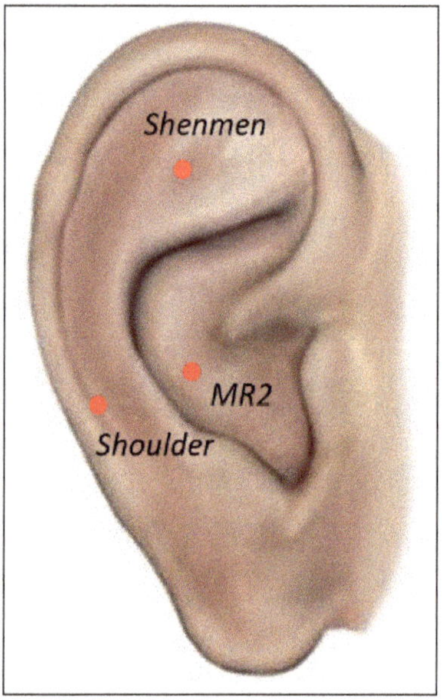

Fig 4.4: Treatment for Acute Shoulder Pain using Ear Seeds

5. Frozen Shoulder

Introduction

- Patient presents with pain in shoulder and restriction of shoulder movements usually in all directions, though it may be more in one or more directions
- It is also known as adhesive capsulitis
- Usually starts gradually but can become chronic.
- May take 6 months to 2 years resolve on its own (without treatment)
- Along with acupressure therapy, frequent exercise (of the shoulder joint) for a short interval (1 - 2 min), 6-8 times a day is necessary for enhancing recovery.

For this condition, bleeding supported by tube application, acupoints and combination therapy gave good results.

Please refer to the Mode of Treatment details and watch the accompanying video from the 'Basic Concepts Chapter' before proceeding for specific protocols described ahead.

Frozen Shoulder - Tube

- Roll Jimmy over the Area of the affected shoulder region in Insect CR of index or any other finger.
- Identify the tender CR point and apply a hollow plastic tube with an adhesive tape in the effective direction (usually vertical at the CR point).
- The CR point which is tender can be either on the dorsal or lateral aspect of the finger.
- Re-examine the pain and ask the patient to move the affected part after 2-3 minutes of tube placement.
- If there is some definite relief after applying the tube (>10%), then retain the tube in that position for 36 - 48 hours, its position must be well secured by an additional Band-aid-like tape. (It should neither be too tight to cause extra pressure nor too loose to move the tube from its place.)
- Displacement of the tube can decrease or even nullify the effect.
- Once removed, it must be reapplied for 8-10 hours every day, at the exact same location, until the problem completely disappears.

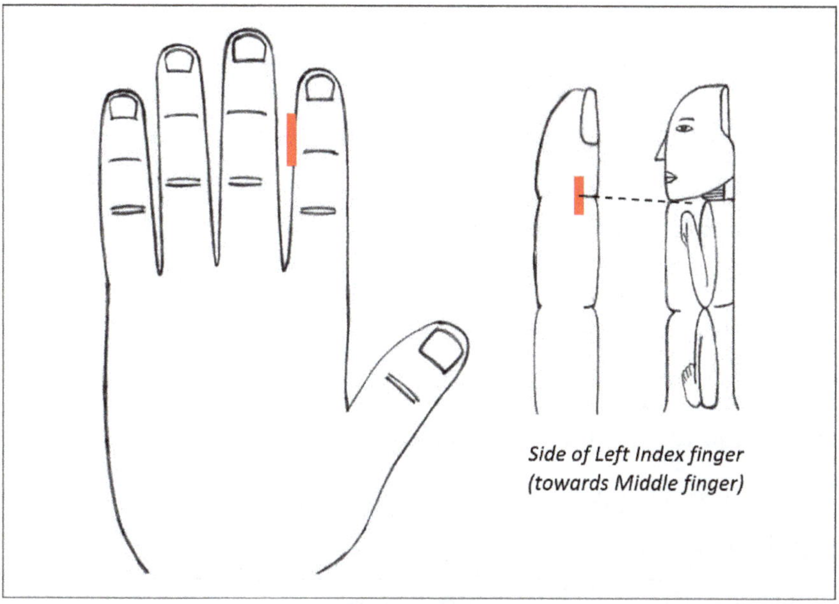

Fig 5.1: Treatment for Left Frozen Shoulder using Insect CR on Left Hand

Frozen Shoulder - Acupoints

- Stimulate the following points by transferring pressure with a jimmy on the Byol meridians of the same side hand as that of the frozen shoulder.
- These points are: GB34, ST45, LI4, LI10, ST38 R (on the opposite hand) and CR.
- If the pain has not fully disappeared after stimulation with jimmy, then apply moong seeds on the same points with the

germinating part (opening) touching the skin with an adhesive tape.

- On the first day, ask the patient to press these seeds 2 hourly for 30 times/minute. Remove them in the morning after pressing them again the same way.
- Subsequently, apply fresh seeds every night. Press them 30 times in one minute. Keep them overnight. Press them again after waking up in the morning and then remove the seeds.
- Continue for 2-20 days as required.
- After 20 days, give a break for 1week and then the seeds can be applied again.

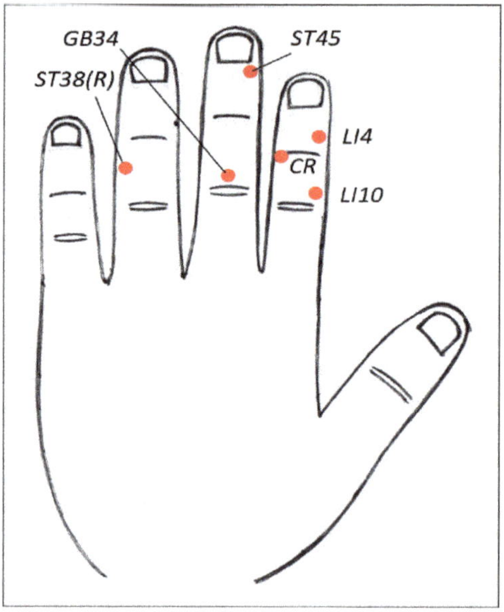

Fig 5.2: Treatment for Left Frozen Shoulder using Byol Meridian

Frozen Shoulder - Bleeding

- Find out the highly tender point on Insect CR with the help of Jimmy.
- The CR point which is tender can be either on the dorsal or lateral aspect of the finger.
- Gently massage the point.
- Clean the area with alcohol (clinical spirit).
- Prick the point with a sterile blood-letting instrument and then bleed 3 to 10 drops of blood under aseptic precautions.
- Apply a hollow plastic tube over the point that is bled. Follow tube protocol for further relief.

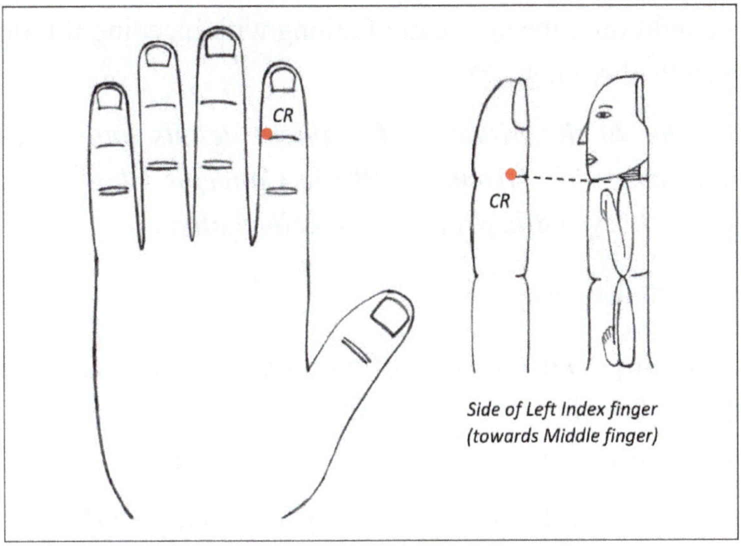

Fig 5.3: Bleeding Treatment for Acute Left Frozen Shoulder using Insect CR

6. Elbow Tendinitis

Introduction

Patient comes with -

- Pain at elbow radiating up & down
- Difficulty in holding things with the affected hand, especially heavy objects.
- Sometimes, it can be associated with swelling.

Tendinitis at elbow can be located at the outer end (Tennis elbow), inner end (Golfer's elbow) or occasionally in the middle.

In this condition, tube application (along with bleeding if required) gave excellent results.

Please refer to the Mode of Treatment details and watch the accompanying video from the 'Basic Concepts Chapter' before proceeding for specific protocols described ahead.

Elbow Tendinitis - Tube

- Roll Jimmy over the Area of the affected elbow region using standard CR along the index finger of the same side or the little finger of the opposite hand.
- Identify the tender CR point and apply a hollow plastic tube with an adhesive tape in the effective direction (usually vertical at the CR point).

- Re-examine the pain and ask the patient to move the affected part after 2-3 minutes of tube placement.
- If there is some definite relief after applying the tube (>10%), then retain the tube in that position for 36 - 48 hours, its position must be well secured by an additional Band-aid-like tape. (It should neither be too tight to cause extra pressure nor too loose to move the tube from its place.)
- Displacement of the tube can decrease or even nullify the effect.
- Once removed, it must be reapplied for 8-10 hours every day, at the exact same location, until the problem entirely disappears.

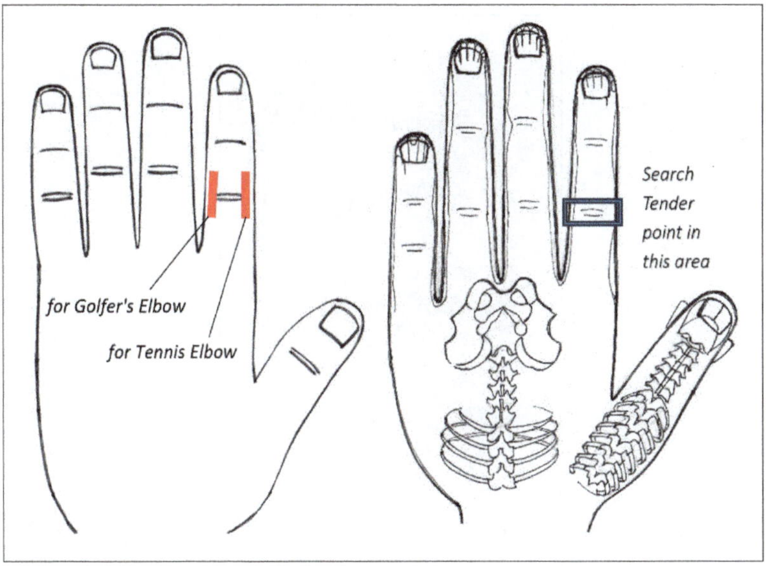

Fig 6.1: Tube Treatment for Left Elbow Tendinitis using Standard CR

Elbow Tendinitis - Ear Seeds

- Check the following ear points for tenderness with the help of a jimmy or point finder.
- The points are Elbow, Shenmen, Muscle Relaxing2 point (MR2).
- Ear seeds are applied at these points after cleaning the ear.
- These are retained for 2-3 weeks.
- The patient should be given instructions on care to be taken.

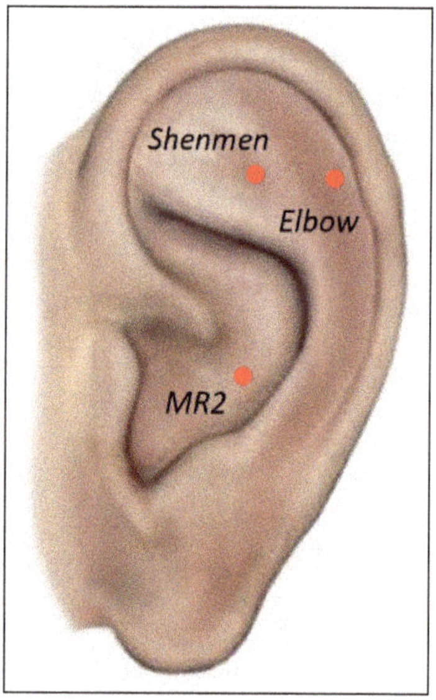

Fig 6.2: Ear seed Treatment for Left Elbow Tendinitis using Ear Seeds

Elbow Tendinitis - Bleeding

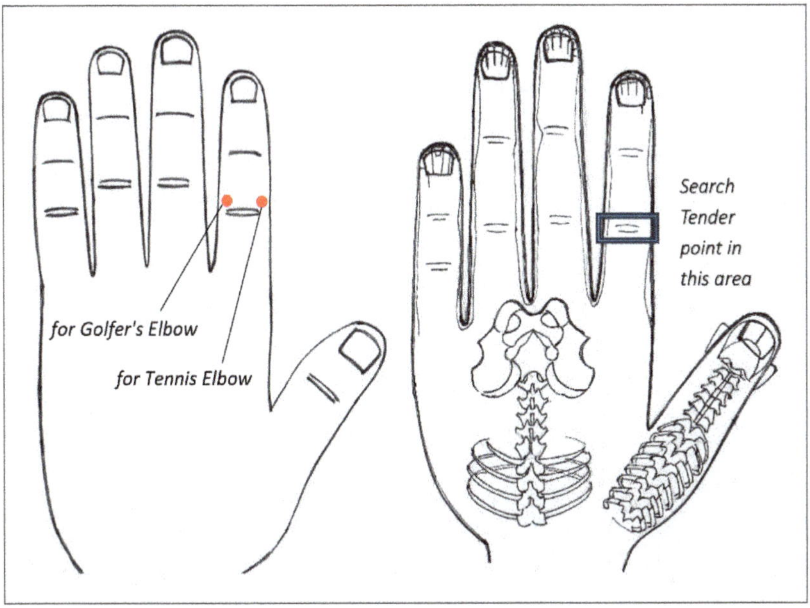

Fig 6.3: Bleeding Treatment for Left Elbow Tendinitis using Standard CR

- Find out the highly tender CR point with the assistance of a jimmy.
- Gently massage the point.
- Clean the area with alcohol (clinical spirit).
- Prick the point with a sterile blood-letting instrument and then bleed 2 to 3 drops of blood with aseptic precautions.
- Apply a hollow plastic tube over the point that is bled. Follow tube protocol for further relief.

Elbow Tendinitis - Acupoints

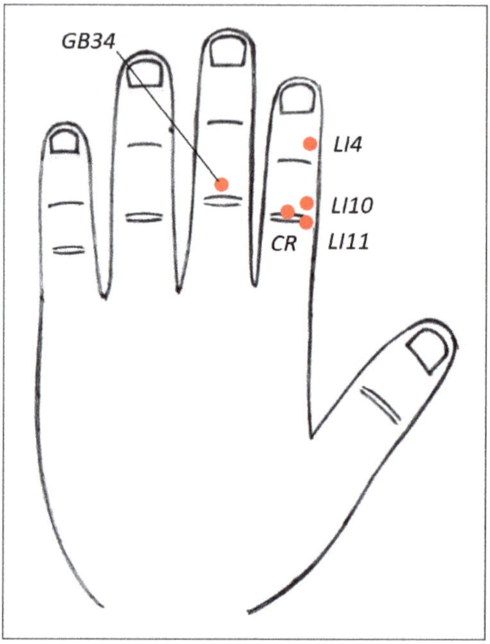

Fig 6.4: Acupoint Treatment for Left Elbow Tendinitis using Byol Meridian

- Stimulate the following points by producing pressure with jimmy on the Byol meridians of the same side hand as that of elbow tendinitis.
- The points are: GB34, Li11, Li4, Li10, CR.
- If the pain has not fully disappeared after stimulation with jimmy, then apply moong seeds on the same points with the

germinating part (opening) touching the skin with an adhesive tape.

- On the first day, ask the patient to press these seeds 2 hourly for 30 times/minute. Remove them in the morning after pressing them again the same way.
- Subsequently, apply fresh seeds every night. Press them 30 times in one minute. Keep them overnight. Press them again after waking up in the morning and then remove the seeds.
- Continue for 2-20 days as required.
- After 20 days, give a break for 1week and then the seeds can be applied again.

7. Wrist & Thumb Pain

Introduction

- A common condition (also known as De Quervain's tenosynovitis) where there is pain on thumb movement & tenderness at the base of the thumb or over a large portion of the thumb. Many a times, wrist movement also gives rise to pain. This makes holding anything or working with that hand difficult.
- It occurs because of inflammation of the tendons of wrist / thumb produced by repetitive motion. The swollen tendons rub against the narrow tunnel they pass through leading to pain which can radiate to the forearm as well. This may develop slowly or suddenly.

For this condition, tube application (along with bleeding if required) gave good results.

Please refer to the Mode of Treatment details and watch the accompanying video from the 'Basic Concepts Chapter' before proceeding for specific protocols described ahead.

Wrist & Thumb Pain - Tube

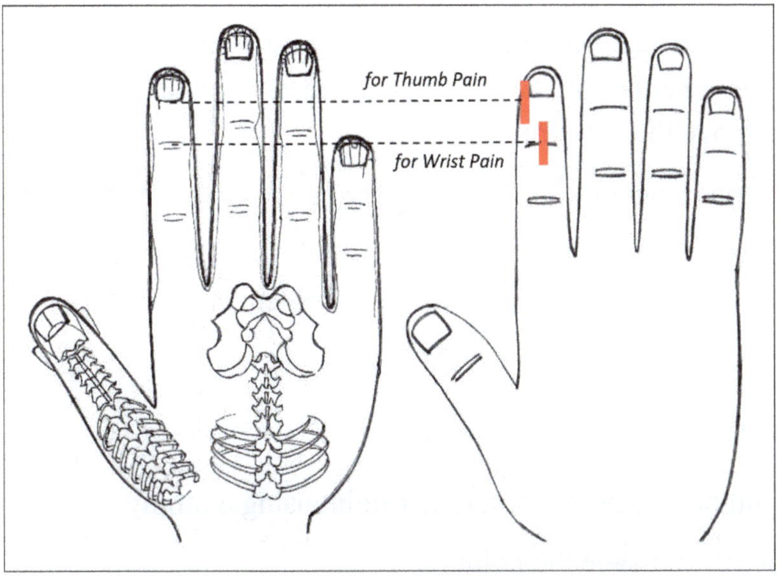

Fig 7.1: Tube Treatment for Right Wrist and Thumb Pain using Standard CR

- Roll Jimmy on the Area of affected part using standard CR along the index finger of the same side or the little finger of the opposite hand.
- Identify the tender CR point and apply a hollow plastic tube with an adhesive tape in the effective direction (usually vertical at the CR point).
- Re-examine the pain and ask the patient to move the affected part after 2-3 minutes of tube placement.

- If there is some definite relief after applying the tube (>10%), then retain the tube in that position for 36 – 48 hours, its position must be well secured by an additional Band-aid-like tape. (It should neither be too tight to cause extra pressure nor too loose to move the tube from its place.)
- Displacement of the tube can decrease or even nullify the effect.
- Once removed, it must be reapplied for 8-10 hours every day, at the exact same location, until the problem entirely disappears.

Wrist & Thumb Pain – Bleeding

- Find out the highly tender CR point using a jimmy.
- Gently massage the point.
- Clean the area with alcohol (clinical spirit).
- Prick the point with a sterile blood-letting instrument and bleed 3 to 10 drops of blood under aseptic precautions.
- Apply a hollow plastic tube over the point that is bled (follow tube protocol) for further relief.

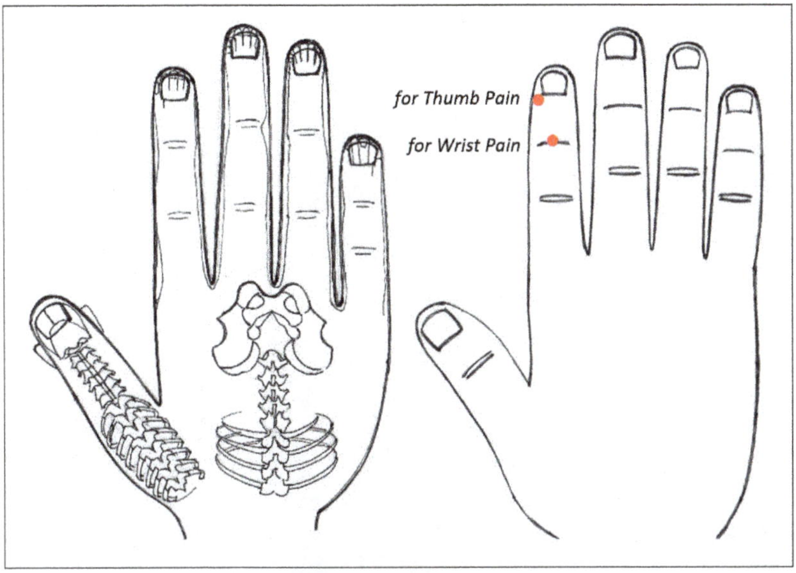

Fig 7.2: Bleeding Treatment for Right Wrist and Thumb Pain using Standard CR

Wrist & Thumb Pain - Ear Seeds

- Check the following ear points for tenderness with the help of jimmy or point finder.
- CR (Wrist/Thumb), Shenmen
- Ear seeds are applied at these points.
- Ear seeds are applied with aseptic precautions.
- These are retained for up to 2 - 3 weeks.

- Patients should be given instructions on care to be taken.

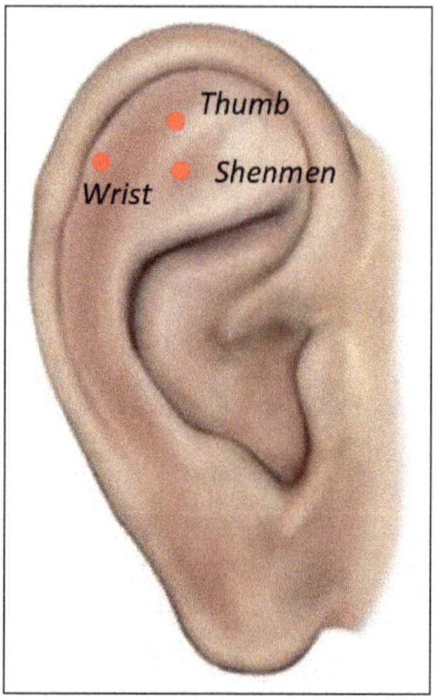

Fig 7.3: Ear Seeds Treatment for Right Wrist and Thumb Pain

8. Compression Neuropathy, Carpal Tunnel

Introduction

It is a condition where the median nerve of the hand gets compressed due to swelling inside the tunnel (made by the bones and the surrounding tissues) as it crosses near the wrist joint.

Similarly, a condition called ulnar neuropathy occurs when the ulnar nerve is compressed as it passes beneath the surface of the skin near the elbow joint.

Compressive neuropathy can occur due to tissue swelling following an arm injury or due to other reasons.

Patient presents with various symptoms:

- Pain in the hand, which at times travels up the forearm towards the shoulder.
- Tingling, numbness, burning and pain in the fingers.
- Weakness, clumsiness, and decreased grip strength of the hand.

In this condition, tube application (along with bleeding if required) was more beneficial.

Please refer to the Mode of Treatment details and watch the accompanying video from the 'Basic Concepts Chapter' before proceeding for specific protocols described ahead.

Carpal Tunnel - Tube

- Roll Jimmy over the Area of affected wrist using standard CR along the index finger of the same side or the little finger of the opposite hand.
- Apply a hollow plastic tube with an adhesive tape in the effective direction (usually horizontal) at the CR point.
- Re-evaluate the pain, numbness and the movement of the hand of the patient after 2-3 minutes of tube placement.
- If there is some definite relief after applying the tube (>10%), then retain the tube in that position for 36 - 48 hours, its position must be well secured by an additional Band-aid-like tape. (It should neither be too tight to cause extra pressure nor too loose to move the tube from its place.)
- Once removed, it must be reapplied for 8-10 hours every day, at the exact same location, until the problem fully disappears.
- Normally, significant relief in pain and numbness is observed immediately and the remaining symptoms including residual pain resolve within 1-3 weeks of tube application.
- Moving the tube from its place can decrease or even nullify the effect.
- **Maintaining the direction of the tube is especially important as a horizontal tube tends to become vertical many a times.** You can also run a thread through the tube to secure the direction. Do make sure that it is not too tight. Apply an adhesive

tape over it, to ensure that it is well secured in the proper direction.

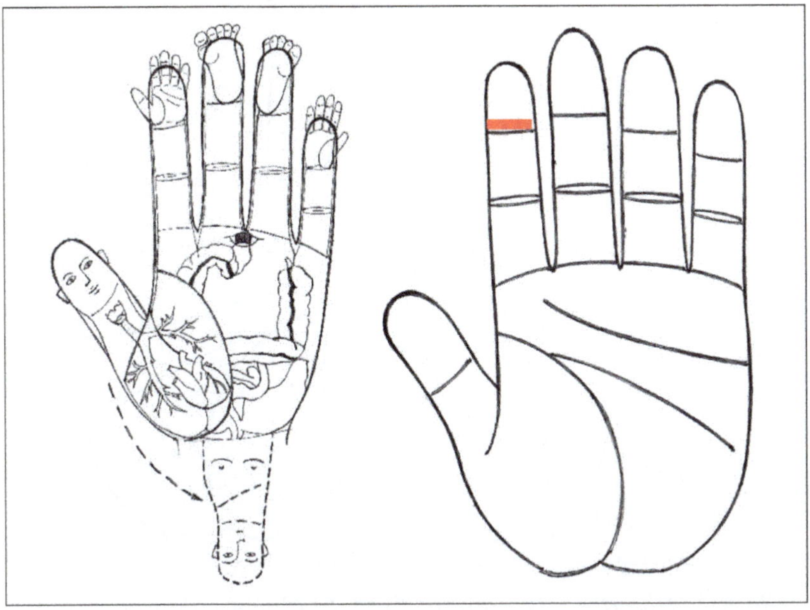

Fig 8.1: Tube Treatment for Left Carpal Tunnel using Standard CR

Carpal Tunnel – Bleeding

- Find out the highly tender CR point with Jimmy.
- Gently massage the point.
- Clean the area with alcohol (clinical spirit).
- Prick the point with a sterile blood-letting instrument and then bleed 8 to 12 drops of blood with aseptic precautions.

- Apply a hollow plastic tube over the point that is bled. Follow tube protocol for further relief.

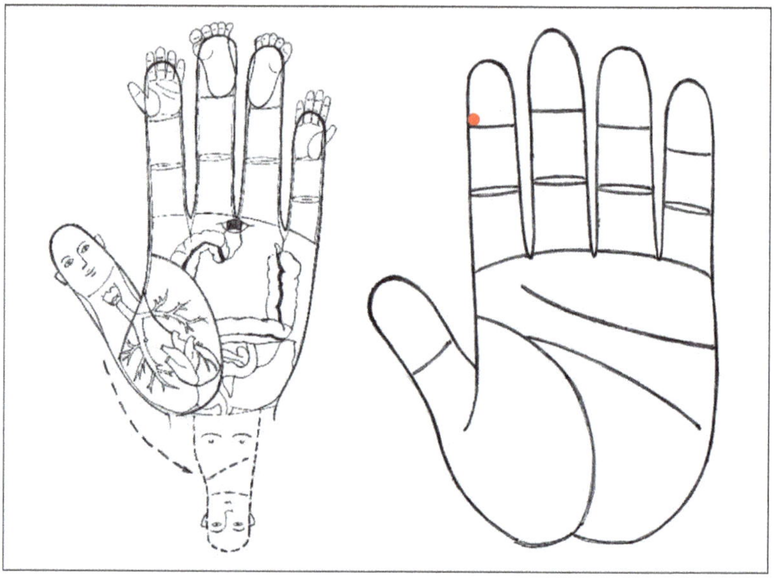

Fig 8.2: Bleeding Treatment for Left Carpal Tunnel using Standard CR

Carpal Tunnel - Acupoints

- Stimulate the following points by providing pressure with jimmy on the Byol meridians of the same side hand as that of carpal tunnel syndrome.
- Li4, Li11 and Ah Shi points (tender points on the area of correspondence).
- If the pain has not fully disappeared after stimulation with jimmy, then apply moong seeds on the same points with the

germinating part (opening) touching the skin with an adhesive tape.

- On the first day, ask the patient to press these seeds 2 hourly for 30 times/minute. Remove them in the morning after pressing them again the same way.
- Subsequently, apply fresh seeds every night. Press them 30 times in one minute. Keep them overnight. Press them again after waking up in the morning and then remove the seeds.
- Continue for 2-20 days as required.
- After 20 days, give a break for 1week and then the seeds can be applied again.

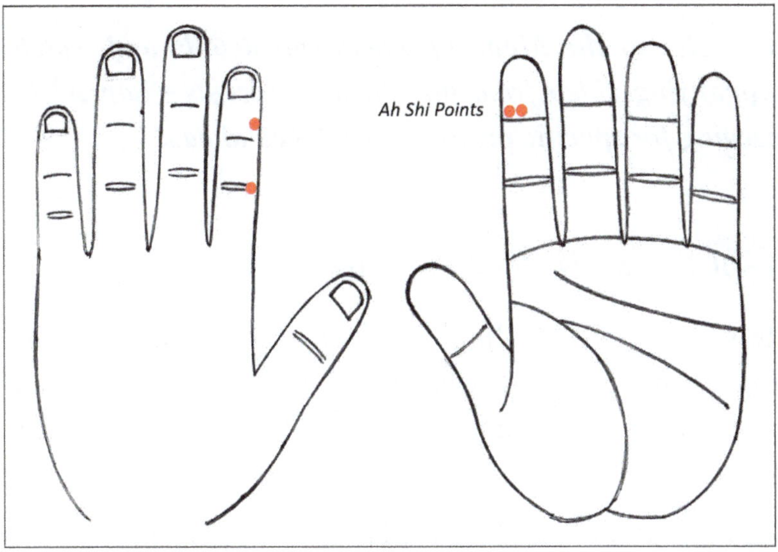

Fig 8.3: Acupoint Treatment for Left Carpal Tunnel using Byol Meridian

9. Acute Upper Extremity Pain along Meridian

Introduction

The patient complains of pain in the outer side (yang side) of upper extremity (UE) with increasing severity over a brief period.

Often, there is a history of repeated action of the upper extremity.

Pain pathway is along the meridian, LI / TW/ SI. The Jing well point located on the meridian is highly tender and can be utilized for therapy.

For this condition, bleeding followed by tube application gave good results.

Please refer to the Mode of Treatment details and watch the accompanying video from the 'Basic Concepts Chapter' before proceeding for specific protocols described ahead.

Acute UE Pain along Meridian - Tube

- Roll Jimmy over the Jing Well points on Byol meridians of the upper extremity using standard CR (LI1, TW1, SI1) along the index finger of the same side or the little finger of the opposite hand.
- Find the most tender Jing Well point and apply a hollow plastic tube with an adhesive tape in a vertical direction at the identified Jing Well point along the meridian.

- Re-evaluate the pain and ask the patient to move the affected part after 2-3 minutes of tube placement.
- If there is some definite relief after applying the tube (>10%), then retain the tube in that position for 36 - 48 hours, its position must be well secured by an additional Band-aid-like tape. (It should neither be too tight to cause extra pressure nor too loose to move the tube from its place.)
- Movement of the tube can decrease or even nullify the effect.
- Once removed, it must be reapplied for 8-10 hours every day, at the exact same location, until the problem fully disappears.

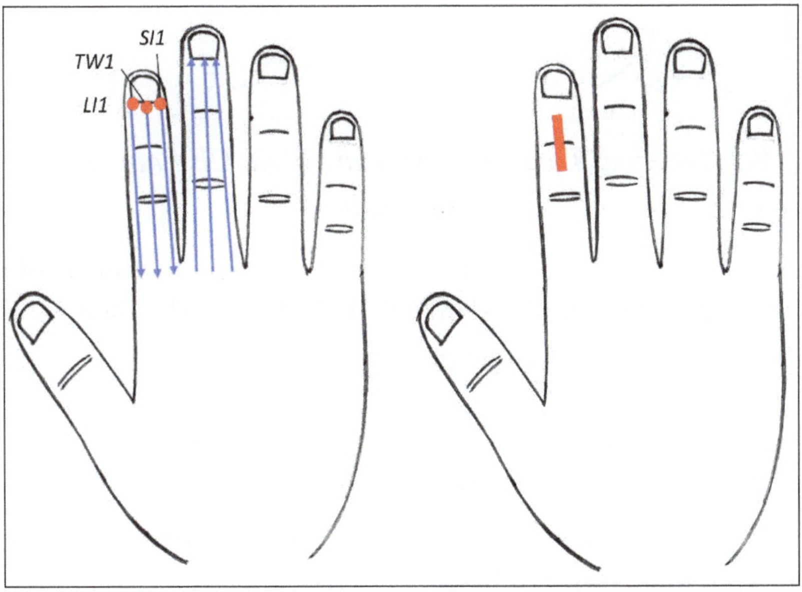

Fig 9.1: Tube Treatment for Acute Left UE Pain along Triple Warmer Meridian

Acute UE Pain along Meridian - Bleeding

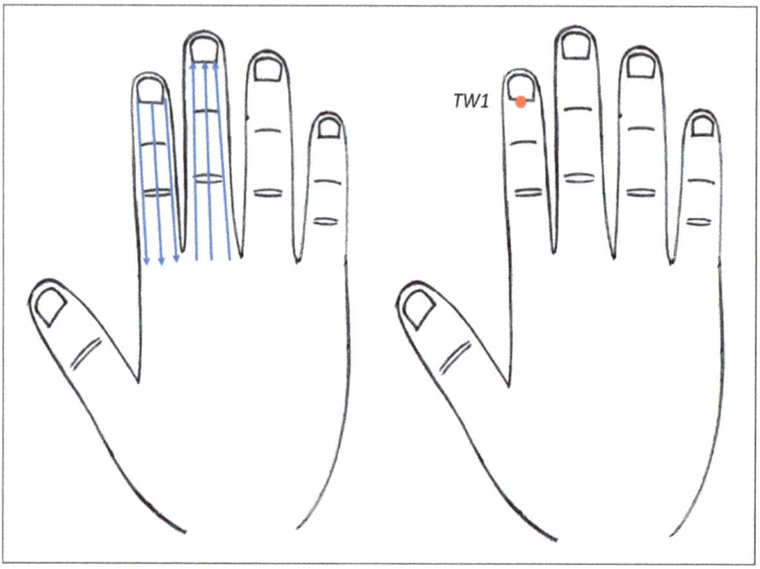

Fig 9.2: Bleeding Treatment for Acute Right UE Pain along TW Meridian

- Roll Jimmy over the Jing Well points on Byol meridians of the upper extremity in Standard CR (LI1, TW1, SI1). Find out the most tender Jing Well point.
- Gently massage the point.
- Clean the area with alcohol (clinical spirit).
- Prick the point with a sterile blood-letting instrument and then bleed 6 to 12 drops of blood with aseptic precautions.
- Apply a hollow plastic tube over the point that is bled. Follow tube protocol for further relief.

Acute UE Pain along Meridian - Acupoints

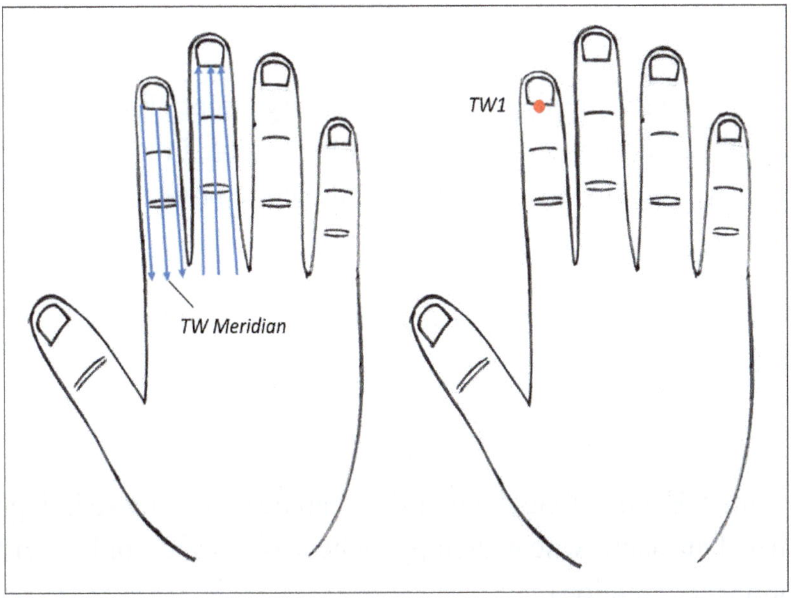

Fig 9.3: Acupoint Treatment for Acute Right UE Pain along TW Meridian

- Roll Jimmy over the Jing Well points on Byol meridians of the upper extremity in Standard CR (LI1, TW1, SI1). Choose the same side hand as that of pain.
- Find out the most tender Jing Well point and stimulate it.
- If the pain has not fully disappeared after stimulation with jimmy, then apply moong seeds on the same points with the germinating part (opening) touching the skin with an adhesive tape.

- On the first day, ask the patient to press these seeds 2 hourly for 30 times/minute. Remove them in the morning after pressing them again the same way.
- Subsequently, apply fresh seeds every night. Press them 30 times in one minute. Keep them overnight. Press them again after waking up in the morning and then remove the seeds.
- Continue for 2-20 days as required.
- After 20 days, give a break for 1 week and then the seeds can be applied again.

Acute UE Pain along Meridian – Wheat Seeds

- Acute UE Pain along the meridian can be treated by sedating the meridian using wheat therapy (wheat seeds are applied in the opposite direction).
- Apply wheat seeds on the specified points such that the germinating end, where the red dot is shown in the figure, must be placed on the skin.
- After applying the wheat seed, ask the patient to wait for 20 minutes. Usually, there is some relief in symptoms during this period. If there is no relief, then at least there should be no aggravation of the symptom or untoward symptom. In such cases the wheat seeds should be removed immediately, and some other method should be tried.
- Every day use fresh wheat seeds.

- For the first 2 days, wheat seeds should be kept for 6-8 hours during the day. The patient is asked to confirm improvement before continuing this treatment. Continue for 2-20 days as required. The duration of the treatment should be tapered when more than 70% pain relief is experienced.
- Treatment should be discontinued once complete relief is obtained.

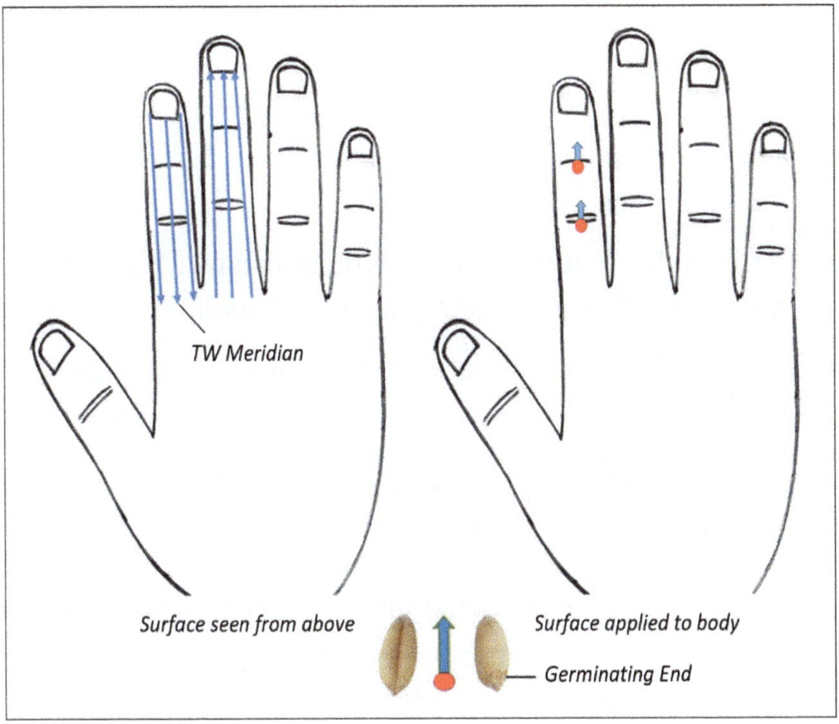

Fig 9.4: Wheat Seed Treatment for Acute Right UE Pain along TW Meridian

10. Trigger Finger

Introduction

- This is quite a common condition and is easy to diagnose.
- In this case, one or more than one finger gets stuck in a bent (flexed) position, and it must be forcibly snapped open making a clicking sound. This movement is painful. It is associated with pain of varying intensity (mild to severe), with or without swelling at the base of the finger on the palm.
- It can slowly progress and cause stiffness in that finger, more so in the morning.
- It occurs due to inflammation in or around the flexor tendon of the finger, affecting its ability to move smoothly.
- Repeated action of that tendon usually predisposes to this condition. Those at risk are women, diabetics, and people whose regular activities strain their hands.
- It may subside on its own, over a period of 1 to 3 months or progress to stiffness. Night splinting, medication to decrease the pain, steroid injections at the site may help decrease the pain but might not retrieve the trapped tendon. Surgery may be required in such a scenario.
- In this condition, tube application (along with bleeding if required) was more beneficial.

Please refer to the Mode of Treatment details and watch the accompanying video from the 'Basic Concepts Chapter' before proceeding for specific protocols described ahead.

Trigger Finger - Tube

- Check which finger or fingers of the patient are involved and look for the tender area or swelling (mild) at the base of the finger on the palm.
- With the help of a jimmy, find the Area of correspondence in standard CR - ventral aspect of the index finger (same side) or the little finger (opposite side).
- Identify the tender CR point and apply a plastic hollow tube with an adhesive tape in the effective direction (usually horizontal at the CR).
- Reassess the pain and ask the patient to move the affected part after 2-3 minutes of tube placement.
- If there is some definite relief after applying the tube (>10%), then retain the tube in that position for 36 - 48 hours, its position must be well secured by an additional Band-aid-like tape. (It should neither be too tight to cause extra pressure nor too loose to move the tube from its place.)
- Movement of the tube can decrease or even nullify the effect.

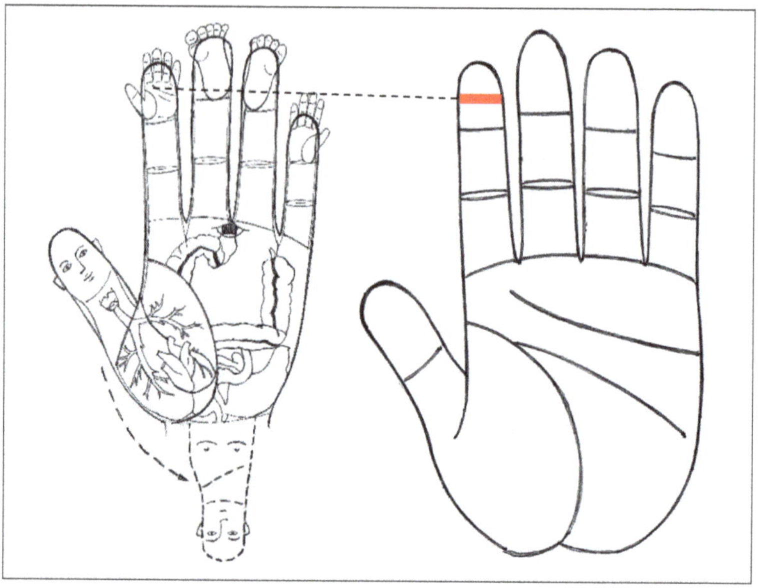

Fig 10.1: Tube Treatment for Left Trigger Finger using Standard CR

- Once removed, it must be reapplied for 8-10 hours every day, at the exact same location, until the problem fully disappears. Typically, substantial relief in pain and movement is observed immediately and the remaining symptoms including residual pain resolve within 1-3 weeks of tube application.
- **Maintaining the direction of the tube is particularly important as a horizontal tube tends to become vertical many a times.** You can also run a thread through the tube to secure the direction. Do make sure that it is not too tight. Apply an adhesive tape over it, to ensure that it is well secured in the proper direction.

Trigger Finger - Bleeding

- Find out the highly tender CR point using Jimmy.
- Gently massage the point.
- Clean the area with alcohol (clinical spirit).
- Prick the point with a sterile blood-letting instrument and then bleed 8 to 12 drops of blood with aseptic precautions.
- Apply a hollow plastic tube over the point that is bled (follow tube protocol) for further relief.

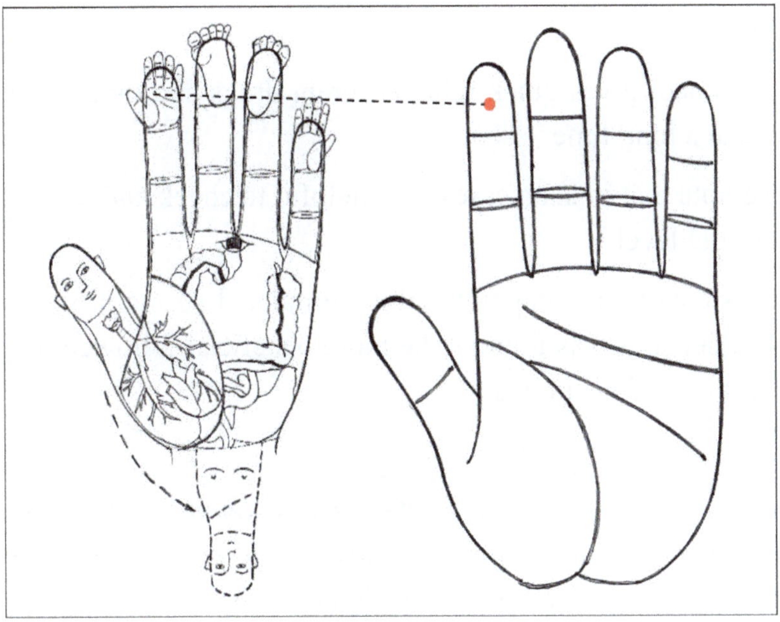

Fig 10.2: Bleeding Treatment for Left Trigger Finger using Standard CR

11. Acute Lower Backache (Acute Lumbosacral Spasm)

Introduction

This is a common and extremely stressful condition where the patient experiences sudden stiffness in the back and is not able to move at all or has great difficulty moving.

Acute Lower Backache without any known cause or injury is usually due to muscular spasm or ligament strain.

Patients complain of acute pain in their lower back and trouble moving.

This protocol gives quick relief wherein drugs and other methods may take a long time.

Please note that in such cases, it is helpful to check and correct the Vitamin D level.

For this condition, acupoint GV26 stimulated strongly by Jimmy for 4 -5 seconds was found to be more beneficial followed by tube application and acupoints.

Please refer to the Mode of Treatment details and watch the accompanying video from the 'Basic Concepts Chapter' before proceeding for specific protocols described ahead.

Acute Lower Backache - Tube

- Roll jimmy on the Area of affected back region in Mini CR system of index finger.
- Identify the CR point and apply a small plastic tube with an adhesive tape in the effective direction (usually vertical) at the CR point.
- Review the pain and ask the patient to move the affected part after 2-3 minutes of tube placement.
- If there is some definite relief after applying the tube (>10%), then retain the tube in that position for 36 - 48 hours, its position must be well secured by an additional Band-aid-like tape. (It should neither be too tight to cause extra pressure nor too loose to move the tube from its place).
- Moving or shifting of the tube from its place can decrease or even nullify the effect.
- Once removed, it must be reapplied for 8-10 hours at the same location every day till the problem fully disappears.

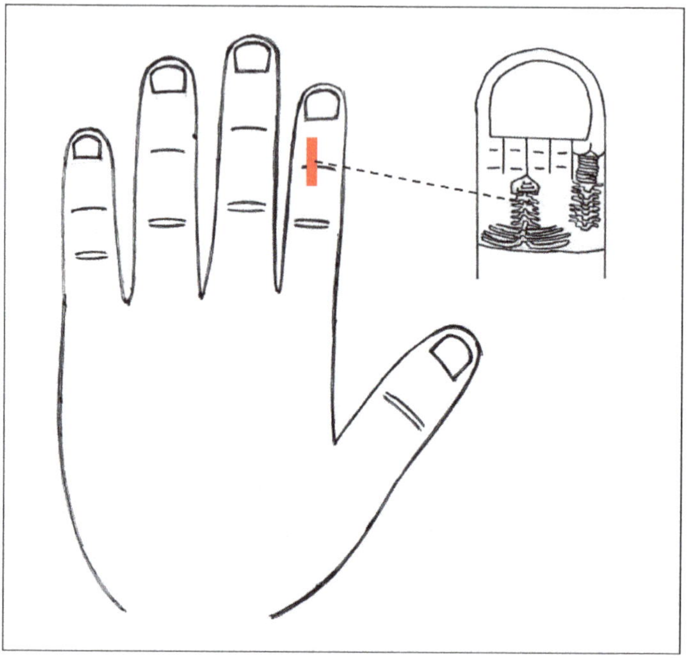

Fig 11.1: Tube Treatment for Acute Lumbosacral Spasm Using Mini CR on Left Index

Acute Lower Backache - Acupoints

- Stimulate and apply pressure on the following points using a jimmy. Choose the same side hand as that of the pain. Alternate moong seed application between left and right hand if the pain is in the center.
- **First try stimulating the point, GV26 for 4-5 seconds with good pressure. This single point can bring relief in most cases.**

- If not, try the following points - GB34, SI3, UB62, GV26, CR.
- If the pain has not fully disappeared after stimulation with jimmy, then apply moong seeds on the same points with the germinating part (opening) touching the skin with an adhesive tape.
- On the first day, ask the patient to press these seeds 2 hourly (30 times in a minute).
- Thereafter, apply only for 8 hours a day till recovery, pressing immediately after application of seeds and at the end of 6-8 hours before removal.
- Every day use fresh seeds. Continue for 1-15 days as required.

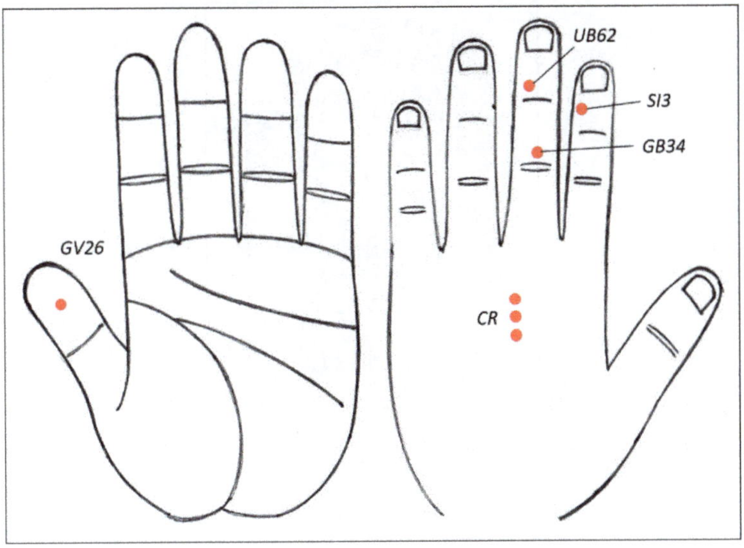

Fig 11.2: Acupoint Treatment for Acute Lumbosacral Spasm Using Byol Meridian

Acute Lower Backache - Ear Seeds

- Check the following points for tenderness with the help of jimmy or point finder.
- The points are CR, Shenmen, Muscle Relaxant point 1 and 2 (MR1 and MR2)
- Ear seeds are applied at these points after cleaning the ear.
- These are retained 2-3 weeks.
- Explain to the patient the essential safety instructions to be followed while using this therapy.

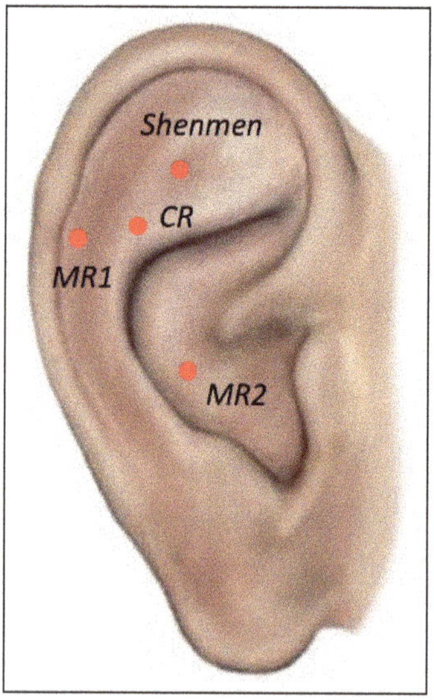

Fig 11.3: Ear Seeds Treatment for Acute Lumbosacral Spasm

Acute Lower Backache - Bleeding

- With the help of Jimmy, find out the highly tender CR point in Mini CR system.
- Gently massage the point.
- Clean the area with alcohol (clinical spirit).
- Prick the point with a sterile blood-letting instrument and then bleed 4 to 10 drops of blood with aseptic precautions.
- This bleeding method is especially useful when there is a history of an injury or sudden jerk in the back.
- Apply a hollow plastic tube over the point that is bled. Follow tube protocol for further relief.

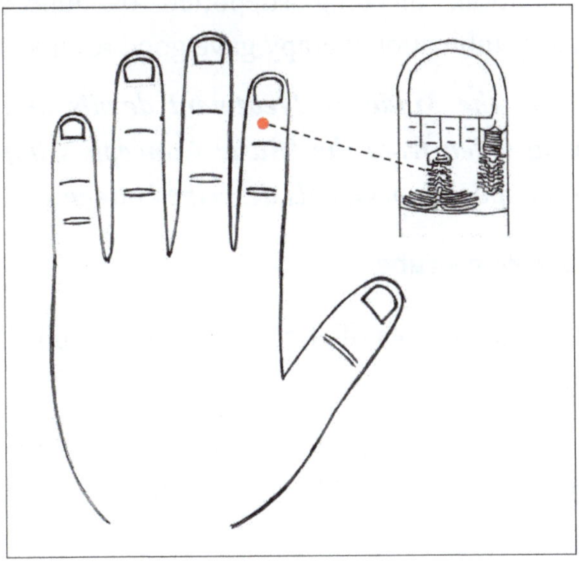

Fig 11.4: Bleeding Treatment for Acute Lumbosacral Spasm Using Mini CR

12. Acute Lumbar Pain

Introduction

Patient comes with a history of pain in the region above the buttock (around the iliac crest). It usually presents acutely but can be long standing in some cases.

It occurs due to muscle spasm after some odd movement or being in one position for a long time.

This may cause problems while walking, bending, or sleeping on that side. Turning and moving around in the bed becomes difficult.

For this condition, bleeding supported by tube application, acupoints and combination therapy gave good results.

Please refer to the Mode of Treatment details and watch the accompanying video from the 'Basic Concepts Chapter' before proceeding for specific protocols described ahead.

Acute Lumbar Pain - Tube

- Roll jimmy on the Area of affected region in Mini CR system of index finger.
- Identify the tender CR point and apply a small plastic tube with an adhesive tape in the effective direction (usually horizontal) at the CR point.
- Review the pain and ask the patient to move the affected part after 2-3 minutes of tube placement.

- If there is some definite relief after applying the tube (>10%), then retain the tube in that position for 36 – 48 hours, its position must be well secured by an additional Band-aid-like tape. (It should neither be too tight to cause extra pressure nor too loose to move the tube from its place).
- Moving of tube from its place can decrease or even nullify the effect.
- Once removed, it must be reapplied for 8-10 hours at the same location every day till the problem fully disappears.

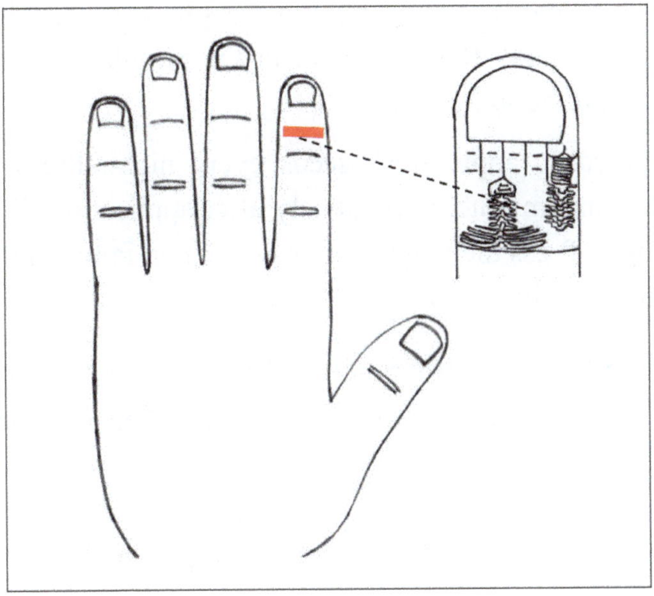

Fig 12.1: Tube Treatment for Left Lumbar Pain Using Mini CR on Left Index

Acute Lumbar Pain - Acupoints

- Stimulate the following points by giving pressure with a jimmy on the Byol meridians of the same side hand as that of the pain.
- These points are GB34, SI3, UB62, CR (Red area).
- If the pain has not fully disappeared after stimulation with jimmy, then apply moong seeds on the same points with the germinating part (opening) touching the skin with an adhesive tape.
- On the first day, ask the patient to press these seeds 2 hourly for 30 times/minute. Remove them in the morning after pressing them again the same way.
- Subsequently, apply fresh seeds every night. Press them 30 times in one minute, immediately after application. Keep them overnight. Press them again after waking up in the morning and then remove the seeds.
- Continue for 2-20 days as required.
- After 20 days, give a break for 1week and then the seeds can be applied again.

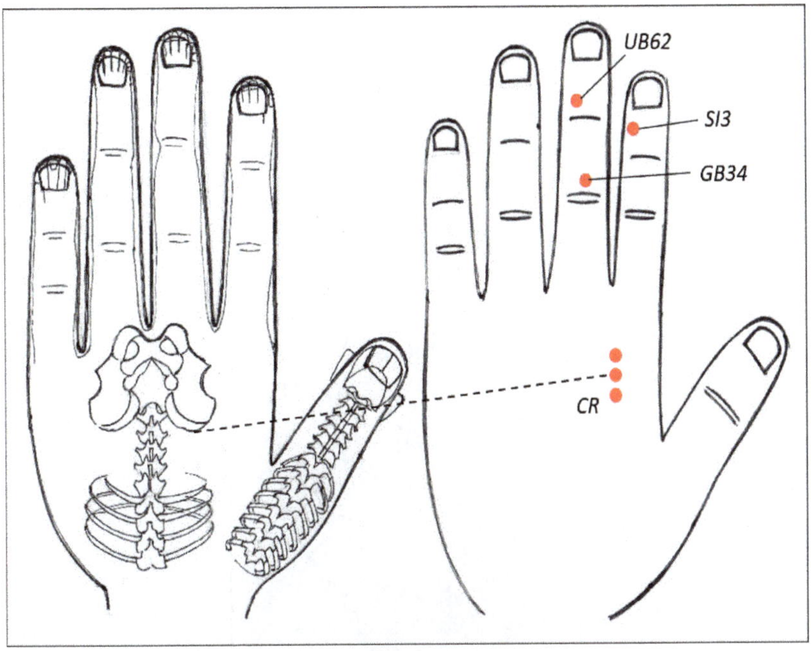

Fig 12.2: Acupoint Treatment for Left Lumbar Pain Using Standard CR

Acute Lumbar Pain – Ear Seeds

- Check the following ear points for tenderness with the help of a jimmy or point finder.
- The points are CR, Shenmen, Muscle Relaxant point1 (MR1).
- Ear seeds are applied at these points after cleaning the ear.
- These are retained for 2-3 weeks.

- The patient should be given instructions on the basic care to be taken.

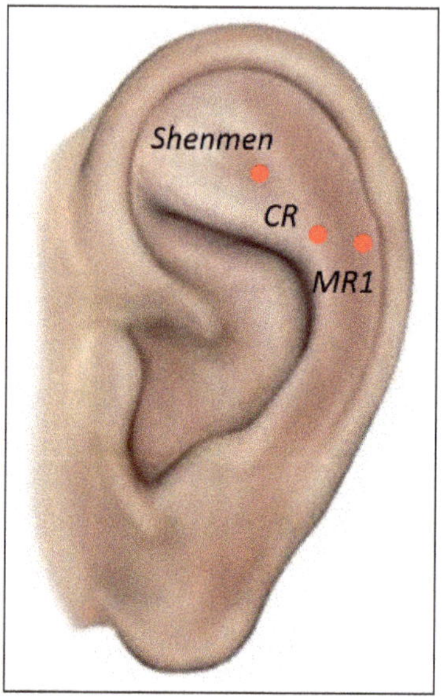

Fig 12.3: Ear Seed Treatment for Left Lumbar Pain

13. Chronic Backache

Introduction

- Chronic backache is a frequent condition, which cannot be attributed to a certain cause even after multiple investigations.
- The patient does not experience much relief even after frequent visits to the doctor or trying out various therapies. This persists despite correcting the Vitamin D level and ruling out osteoporosis. In such a scenario, ligament strain, deep muscle spasm, weakness in the ligaments or muscles may be the cause.
- Many such cases have responded very well to this protocol.
- Along with acupressure therapy, back and abdominal exercises should be done regularly under proper guidance for enhancing recovery.
- Pranayama also helps in any chronic pain and should be advised.

In this condition, tube application and acupoints with seeds have been found to be more effective.

Please refer to the Mode of Treatment details and watch the accompanying video from the 'Basic Concepts Chapter' before proceeding for specific protocols described ahead.

Chronic Backache – Tube

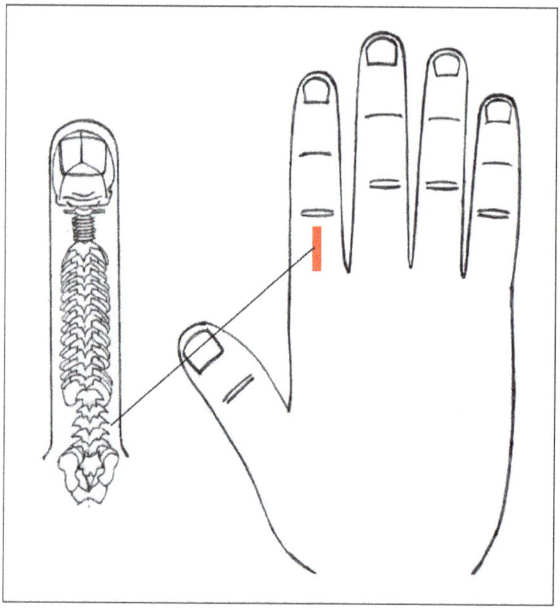

Fig 13.1: Tube Treatment for Chronic Backache using Insect CR

- Roll Jimmy over the Area of the affected back region in Insect CR of index or any other finger to locate the tender point.
- Apply a small plastic tube with adhesive tape in the effective direction of tenderness (usually vertical) at the CR point.
- Re-examine the pain and ask the patient to move the affected part after 2-3 minutes of tube placement.
- If there is some definite relief after applying the tube (>10%), then retain the tube in that position for 36 – 48 hours, its

position must be well secured by an additional Band-aid-like. (It should neither be too tight to cause extra pressure nor too loose to move the tube from its place.)

- Displacement of the tube can decrease or even nullify the effect.
- Once removed it must be reapplied for 8-10 hours every day, at the exact same location, until the problem completely disappears.

Chronic Backache - Acupoints

- Stimulate the following points by giving pressure with jimmy on the Byol meridians. Choose the same hand as the side of pain or use both hands alternately if the pain is in the center.
- These points are CV4, CV6, GV14, UB11, UB23, GV4, K3, K6, K7, SI3, and UB62 on both hands, alternatingly.
- In addition to the above Acupoints, seeds are also applied on the Insect CR of any convenient finger for further benefit (Refer Figure - Insect CR on Ring finger).
- If the pain has not fully disappeared after stimulation with jimmy, then apply moong seeds on the same points with the germinating part (opening) touching the skin with an adhesive tape.
- On the first day, ask the patient to press these seeds 2 hourly for 30 times/minute. Remove them in the morning after pressing them again the same way.

- Subsequently, apply fresh seeds every night. Press them 30 times in one minute. Keep them overnight. Press them again after waking up in the morning and then remove the seeds.
- Continue for 2-20 days as required.
- Alternate moong seed application between left and right hand if the pain is in the center.
- After 20 days, give a break for 1week and then the seeds can be applied again.

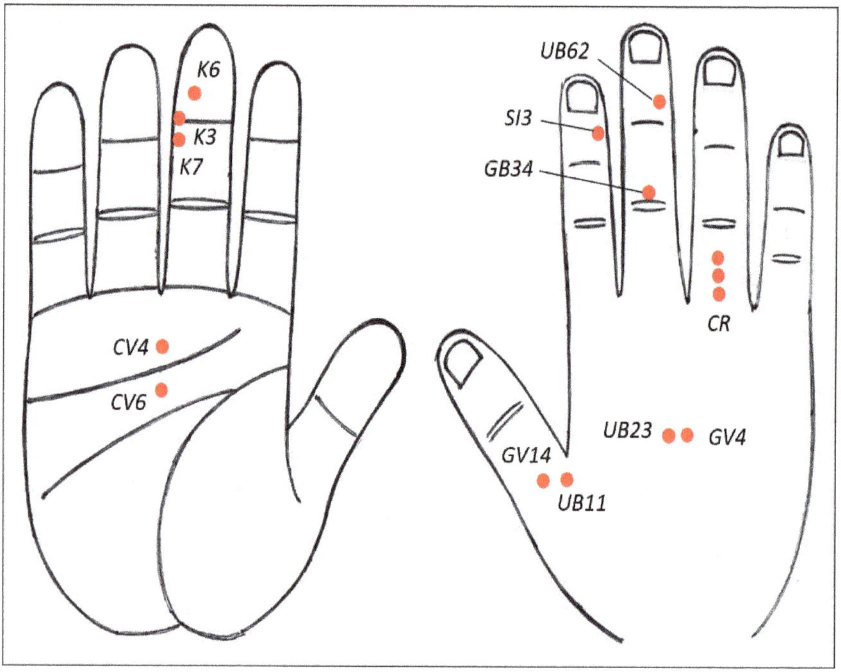

Fig 13.2: Acupoint Treatment for Chronic Backache using Byol Meridian on Right Hand

Chronic Backache - Bleeding

- Identify the highly tender CR point on index finger with the help of Jimmy in Insect CR system.
- Gently massage the point.
- Clean the area with alcohol (clinical spirit).
- Prick the point with a sterile blood-letting instrument like lancet/needle and bleed 1 to 5 drops of blood with aseptic precautions.
- Apply a hollow plastic tube over the point that is bled (follow tube protocol) for further relief.

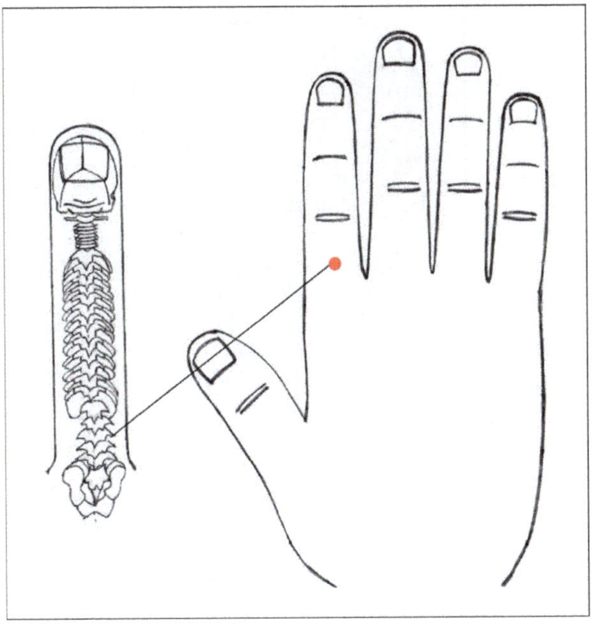

Fig 13.3: Bleeding Treatment for Chronic Backache

Chronic Backache - Ear Seeds

- Check the following ear points for tenderness with the help of jimmy or point finder.
- These points are Shenmen, Muscle Relaxant1 (MR1), Muscle Relaxant2 (MR2), Kidney and CR.
- Ear seeds are applied at these points after cleaning the ear.
- These are retained for 2-3 weeks.
- The patient should be given instructions on care to be taken.

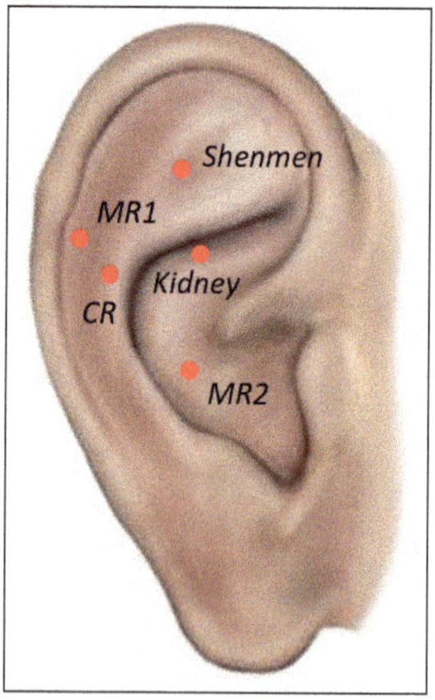

Fig 13.4: Ear seed Treatment for Chronic Backache

14. Tailbone Pain (Coccydynia)

Introduction

This condition represents the pain which occurs in and around the tailbone (coccyx) leading to difficulty in sitting, especially on a firm / hard surface and for a longer duration.

It may begin post injury or prolonged sitting over an unpadded seat (e.g.: cycling). This condition tends to become chronic and does not have an easy solution.

This protocol is worth trying as the patient responds very well and quickly. In this condition, ear seeds give instant relief. If not, wheat seed therapy may be attempted.

Please refer to the Mode of Treatment details and watch the accompanying video from the 'Basic Concepts Chapter' before proceeding for specific protocols described ahead.

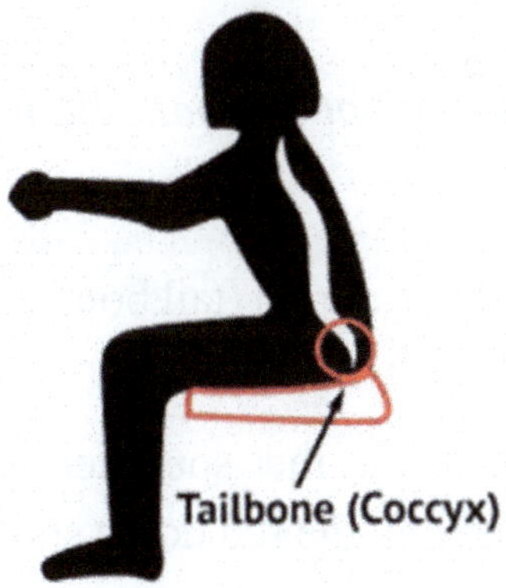

Fig 14: Tailbone Pain

Tailbone Pain – Wheat Seeds

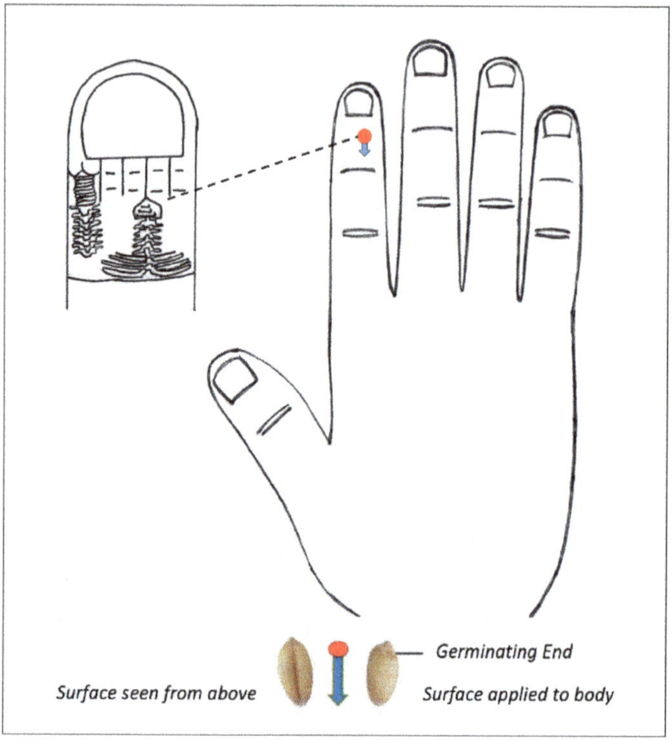

Fig 14.1: Treatment for Tailbone Pain Using Mini CR

- Identify the painful CR region (tail bone CR) in Mini CR system of any finger. You case use Jimmy for this purpose.
- Apply wheat seeds on the specified points such that the germinating end, where the red dot is shown in the figure, must be placed on the skin.

- After applying the wheat seed, ask the patient to wait for 20 minutes. Usually there is some relief in symptoms during this period. If there is no relief, then at least there should be no aggravation of the symptom or untoward symptom. In such cases the wheat seeds should be removed immediately, and some other method should be tried.
- For the first 2 days, wheat seeds should be kept for 8-12 hours during the day. The patient is asked to confirm improvement before continuing this treatment.
- Every day use fresh wheat seeds.
- Continue for 2-20 days as required. The duration of the treatment should be tapered when more than 70% pain relief is experienced.
- Treatment should be discontinued once complete relief is obtained.

Tailbone Pain – Acupoints

- Stimulate the affected CR points by giving pressure with jimmy on the Mini CR and Standard CR.
- If the pain has not fully disappeared after stimulation with jimmy, then apply moong seeds on the same points with the germinating part (opening) touching the skin with an adhesive tape.

- On the first day, ask the patient to press these seeds 2 hourly for 30 times/minute. Remove them in the morning after pressing them again the same way.
- Subsequently, apply fresh seeds every night. Press them 30 times in one minute, immediately after application. Keep them overnight. Press them again after waking up in the morning and then remove the seeds.
- Continue for 2-20 days as required.
- After 20 days, give a break for 1week and then the seeds can be applied again.

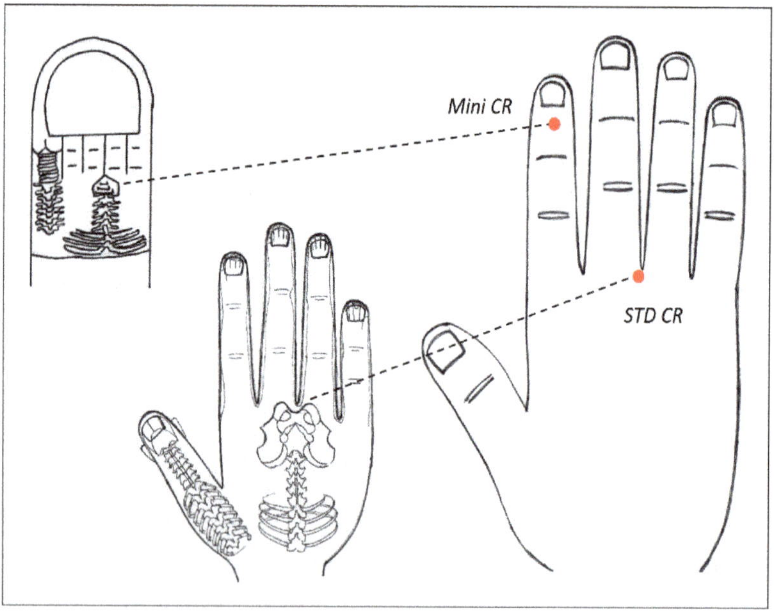

Fig 14.1: Acupoint Treatment for Tailbone Pain Using Mini CR and Standard CR

Tailbone Pain - Ear Seeds

- Check the following ear points for tenderness with the help of jimmy or point finder.
- The points are Muscle Relaxant1, CR.
- Ear seeds are applied at these points after cleaning the ear.
- These are retained for 2-3 weeks.
- The patient should be given instructions on the basic care to be taken.

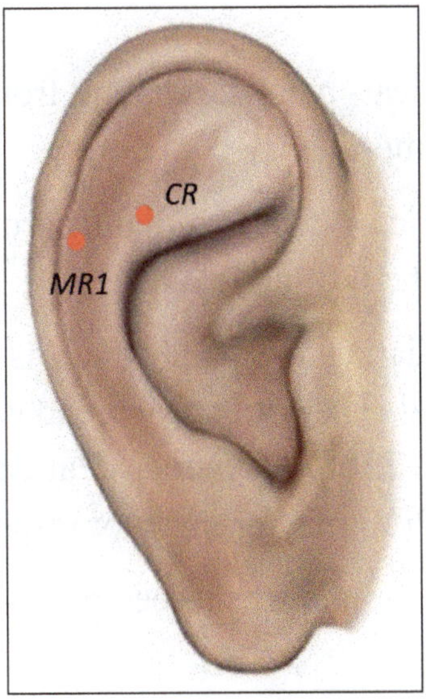

Fig 14.3: Ear Seed Treatment for Tailbone Pain

15. Sciatica

Introduction

The term 'Sciatica' is not clearly defined and is often used inconsistently by clinicians and patients.

Patients complain of radiating pain from the lateral side of the leg (hip region) or back side of the leg (buttock region). The pain radiates from above and moves downwards along that line (back/lateral side) towards the foot.

The Sciatica is classified as follows based on the location of the pain.

1. UB type Sciatica - pain is radiating from the back of the leg along the UB meridian.
2. GB type Sciatica - pain is radiating from the lateral side of the leg along the GB meridian.

In this protocol, radiating leg pain which is not associated with backache is addressed. The patient can bend easily and the straight leg raising test (SLRT) is free. Patients with prolapsed intervertebral disk (PID) may or may not respond to this protocol.

For this condition, we found wheat seed protocol and acupoint with seeds more useful.

Please refer to the Mode of Treatment details and watch the accompanying video from the 'Basic Concepts Chapter' before proceeding for specific protocols described ahead.

Sciatica – Tube

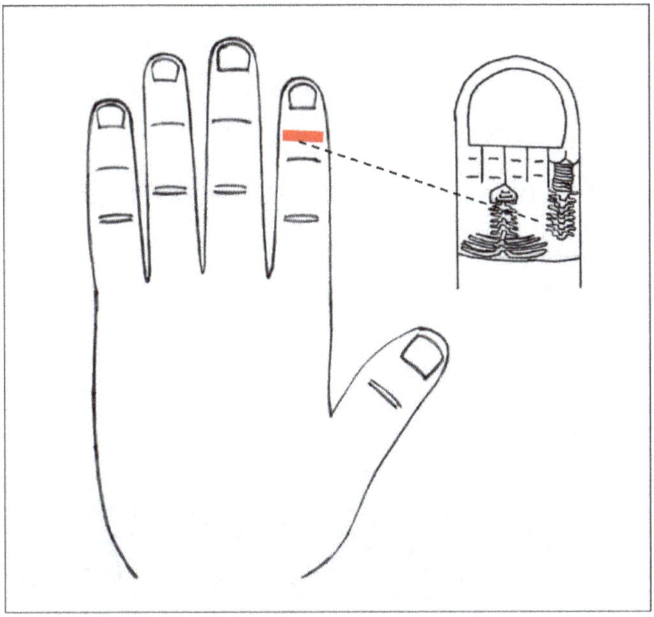

Fig 15.1: Tube Treatment for Left Sciatica using Mini CR

- Roll Jimmy over the Area of the affected region in Mini CR of Index finger or any other finger to locate the tender point.
- Usually, the most tender point is obtained on lateral side of the finger as shown in the figure.
- Apply a hollow plastic tube with an adhesive tape in the effective direction at the CR point (usually horizontal).
- Re-evaluate the pain and ask the patient to move the affected part after 2-3 minutes of tube placement.

- If there is some definite relief after applying the tube (>10%), then retain the tube in that position for 36 - 48 hours, its position must be well secured by an additional Band-aid-like tape. (It should neither be too tight to cause extra pressure nor too loose to move the tube from its place.)
- Displacement of the tube can decrease or even nullify the effect.
- Once removed, it must be reapplied for 8-10 hours every day, at the exact same location, until the problem entirely disappears.

Sciatica - Acupoints

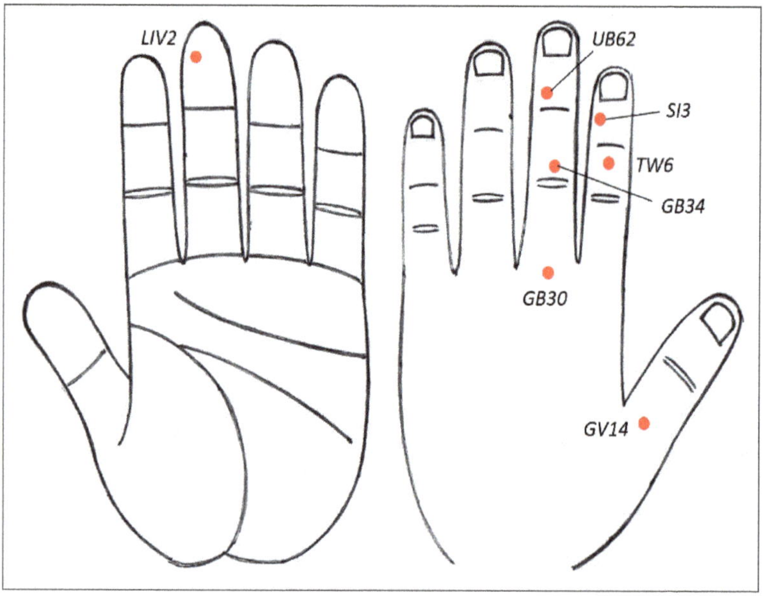

Fig 15.2: Acupoint Treatment of Left Sciatica using Byol Meridian

- Stimulate the following points by giving pressure with a jimmy on the Byol meridians of the same side hand as that of the pain.
- These points are UB62, GB34, GB30, SI3, TW6, LIV2 and GV14.
- If the pain has not fully disappeared after stimulation with jimmy, then apply moong seeds on the same points with the germinating part (opening) touching the skin with an adhesive tape.
- On the first day, ask the patient to press these seeds 2 hourly for 30 times/minute. Remove them in the morning after pressing them again the same way.
- Subsequently, apply fresh seeds every night. Press them 30 times in one minute. Keep them overnight. Press them again after waking up in the morning and then remove the seeds.
- Continue for 2-20 days as required.
- After 20 days give rest for 1week and then seeds can be applied again.

Sciatica - Ear Seeds

- Check the following ear points for tenderness with the help of a jimmy or point finder.
- The points are TW, GB, Sciatica, CR, Shenmen and MR1.
- Ear seeds are applied at these points after cleaning the ear.
- These are retained for 2-3 weeks.

- The patient should be given instructions on care to be taken.

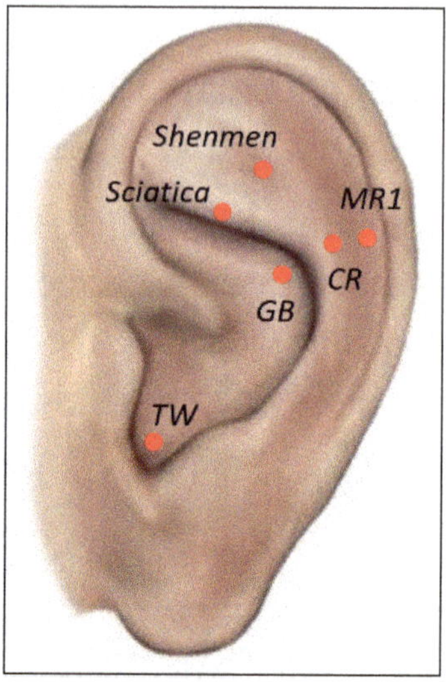

Fig 15.3: Ear Seed Treatment for Left Sciatica

Sciatica – Wheat Seeds

- This method can be used first if there is a history of pain that increases over a brief time or is recurring. In 2 patients whose gall bladder was removed, this method has worked very well.
- Apply wheat seeds on the specified points such that the germinating end, where the red dot is shown in the figure, must be placed on the skin (depending upon the pain - UB type or GB type). This is to sedate that particular meridian.
- After applying the wheat seed, ask the patient to wait for 20 minutes. Usually there is some relief in symptoms during this period.

- If there is no relief, then at least there should be no aggravation of the symptom or untoward symptom. In such cases the wheat seeds should be removed immediately, and some other method should be tried.
- For the first 2 days, wheat seeds should be kept for 8-12 hours during the day. The patient is asked to confirm improvement before continuing this treatment.
- Every day use fresh wheat seeds.
- If there is no response, then move to other methods.

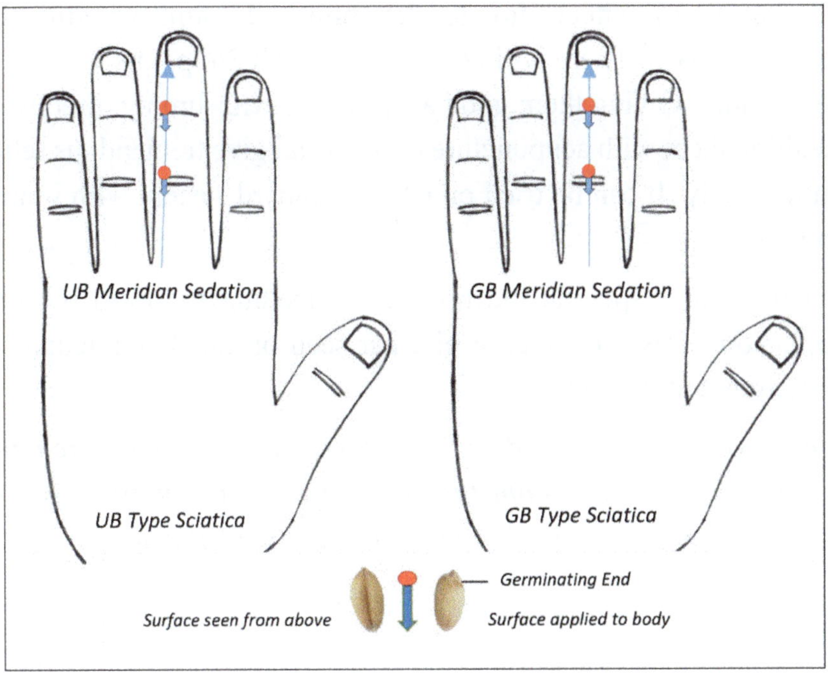

Fig 15.4: Wheat Seed Treatment for Left UB / GB type Sciatica

16. Acute Knee Pain

Introduction

This is commonly due to muscular spasm or ligament strain following a fall or some kind of blunt trauma. Patients complain of acute pain in the knee region, either the front or back. Swelling may be present.

Note: IN SUDDEN ONSET SEVERE KNEE PAIN, where the patient cannot walk or bend the knee (and was walking normally till that time), **check for tender points in and around the popliteal fossa**. There will be quite a few Ah Shi points which are very tender. Giving them good acupressure with Jimmy directly or needling them with acupuncture needles can give tremendous relief immediately. It can be tried on CR in standard system with jimmy and seeds.

If pain is at a specific location, then bleeding followed by tube application was effective, or else ear seed protocol and acupoints were found to be useful.

Please refer to the Mode of Treatment details and watch the accompanying video from the 'Basic Concepts Chapter' before proceeding with the specific protocol described ahead.

Search for tender points (usually 5-7) in the marked area behind the knee. Give good pressure with blunt jimmy or thumb. Acupuncture needles work best in these cases.

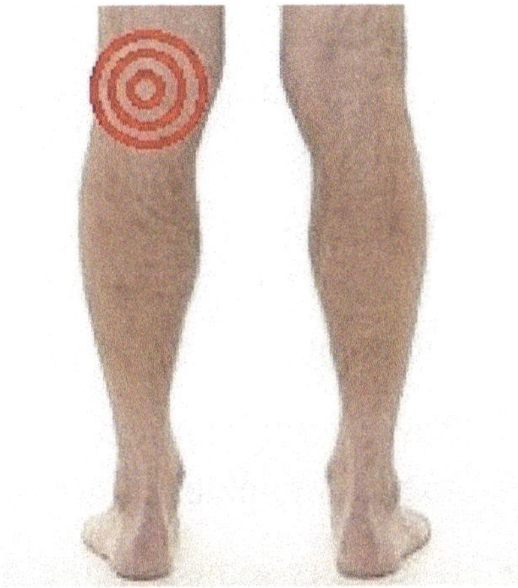

Fig 16: Knee Pain

Acute Knee Pain - Tube

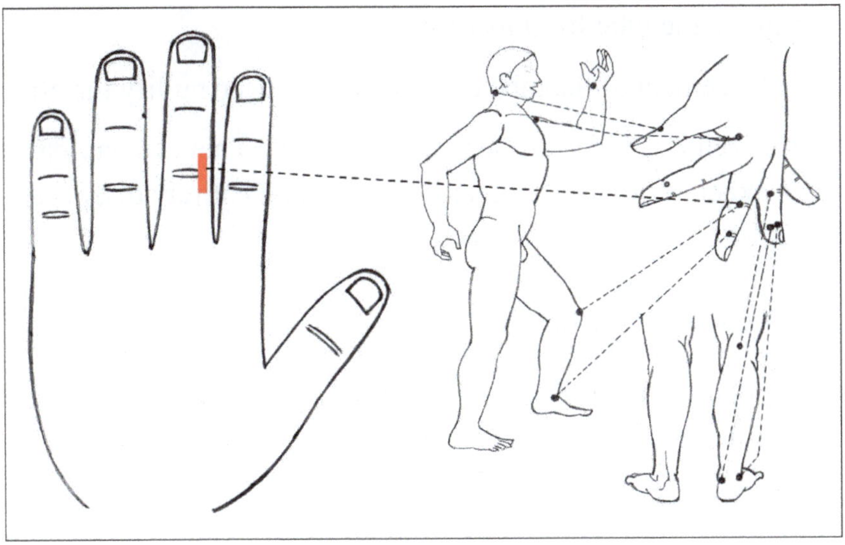

Fig 16.1: Tube Treatment for Left Acute Knee Pain using Standard CR

- Roll Jimmy over the Area of the affected knee in Standard CR along the middle finger of the same hand or on ring finger of the other hand.
- Identify the CR point and apply a hollow plastic tube with adhesive tape in the effective direction (usually vertical) at the CR point.
- Review the pain and ask the patient to move the affected part after 2-3 minutes of tube placement.
- If there is some definite relief after applying the tube (>10%), then retain the tube in that position for 36 – 48 hours, its position must be well secured by an additional Band-aid-like tape. (It should neither be too tight to cause extra pressure nor too loose to move the tube from its place.)
- Displacement of the tube can decrease or even nullify the effect.
- Once removed, it must be reapplied for 8-10 hours every day, at the exact same location, until the problem entirely disappears.

Acute Knee Pain - Acupoints

- Stimulate following points by giving pressure with jimmy on the Byol meridians.
- GB34, ST45, ST36, UB54, LIV2, LIV8

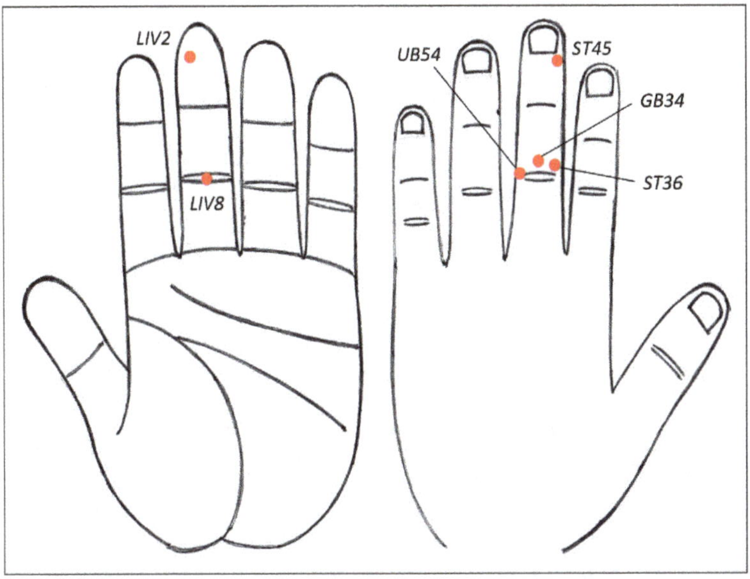

Fig 16.2: Acupoint Treatment for Left Acute Knee Pain using Standard CR

- If the pain has not fully disappeared after stimulation with jimmy, then apply moong seeds on the same points with the germinating part (opening) touching the skin with an adhesive tape.
- On the first day, ask the patient to press these seeds 2 hourly for 30 times/minute. Remove them in the morning after pressing them again the same way.
- Subsequently, apply fresh seeds every night. Press them 30 times in one minute. Keep them overnight. Press them again after waking up in the morning and then remove the seeds.

- Continue for 2-20 days as required.
- After 20 days, give a break for 1week and then the seeds can be applied again.

Acute Knee Pain - Bleeding

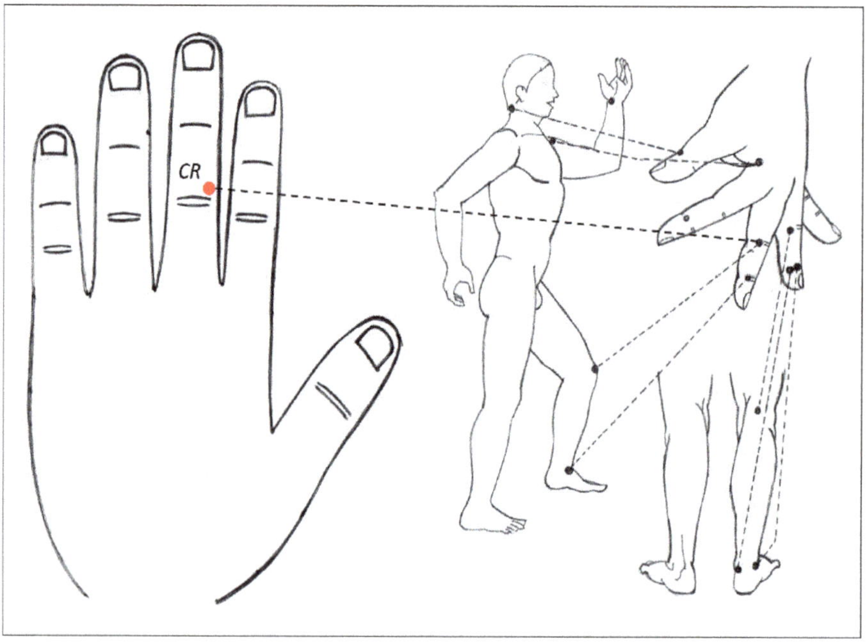

Fig16.3: Bleeding Treatment for Left Acute Knee Pain on Standard CR

- Find out the highly tender point on Standard CR with the help of jimmy.
- Gently massage the point.

- Clean the area with alcohol (clinical spirit).
- Prick the point with a sterile blood-letting instrument and then bleed 8 to 12 drops of blood under aseptic precautions.
- Apply a tube on this point after bleeding (follow Tube protocol) for further relief.
- This method is especially useful if there is a history of injury/ trauma to the knee.

Acute Knee Pain - Tulsi Leaf

- This mode is especially used for cases with swelling around the knee.
- Roll Jimmy in the CR area.
- Apply Tulsi Leaf (non-toxic or any non-irritant fresh green leaf) using adhesive tape in horizontal direction around the first IP joint with stalk towards little finger and rough surface touching the skin (as shown in the figure).
- Keep it in position for nearly 22 hours a day, for 3 days. Change the leaf every day after bath.
- After 3 days, it can be applied every night for 8-10 hours till swelling completely disappears.

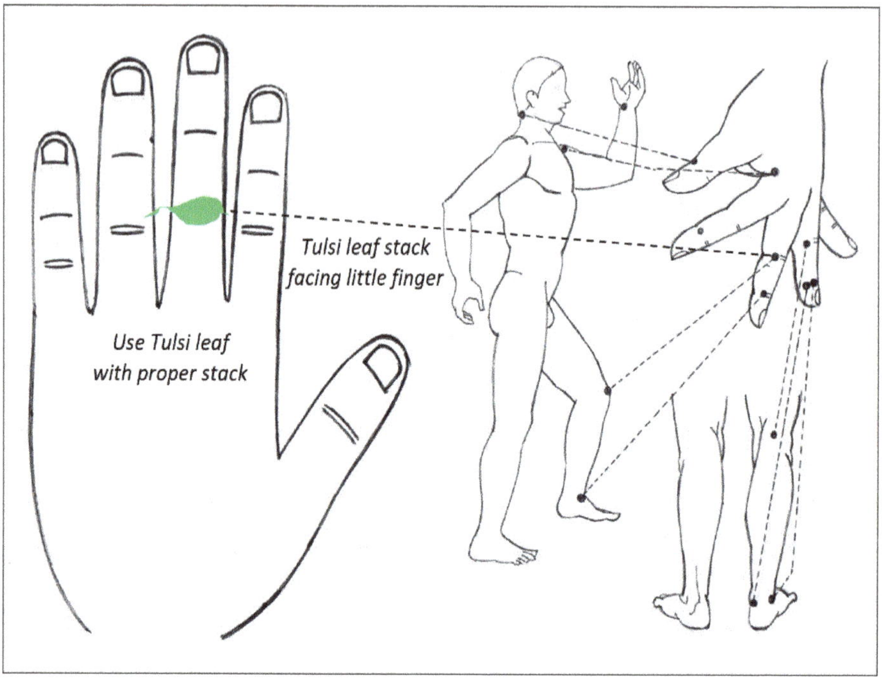

Fig 16.4: Tulsi Leaf Treatment for Left Acute Knee Pain with swelling using Standard CR

Acute Knee Pain - Ear Seeds

- Check the following ear points for tenderness with the help of a jimmy or point finder.
- These points are Knee, Shenmen, Muscle relaxing point 1 and 2 (MR1 and MR2).
- Ear seeds are applied at these points after cleaning the ear.

- These are to be retained for up to 2-3 weeks.
- The patient should be given instructions on care to be taken.

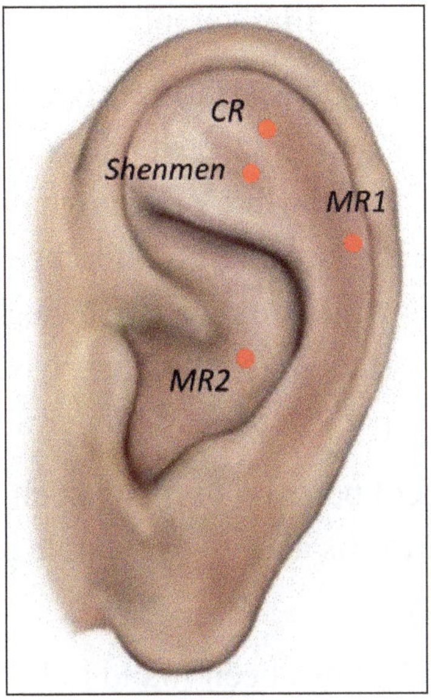

Fig 16.5: Ear Seeds Treatment for Left Acute Knee Pain

17. Chronic Knee Pain

Introduction

Chronic knee pain is a familiar complaint among adults.

It gets associated with Osteoarthritis of the knee which is very prevalent in the older age group. However, other causes of knee pain are also quite common like odd movements, twists, or turns while playing / walking, or running on uneven surfaces, sitting in an odd position, jerks while riding a two-wheeler etc. These causes may result in strain on the ligaments and tissues around the knee leading to pain that is persistent for a longer duration.

The following protocol benefits in many such cases. It can also be tried in early osteoarthritis and gives reliable results. Ear seeds are helpful in these cases.

Application of Tulsi leaf has been found to be useful when there is an associated swelling.

All cases of Chronic Knee Pain are to be treated after a proper diagnosis.

If pain is at specific location, then bleeding followed by tube application was effective, else acupoints with seeds were more beneficial than other methods.

Please refer to the Mode of Treatment details and watch the accompanying video from the 'Basic Concepts Chapter' before proceeding with the specific protocol described ahead.

Chronic Knee Pain - Tube

- Roll Jimmy over the area of affected knee in Standard CR system along the middle finger of the same hand or the ring finger of the opposite hand.
- Identify the tender CR point and apply a hollow plastic tube with adhesive tape in the effective direction (usually vertical) at the CR point.
- Re-examine the pain and ask the patient to move the affected part after 2-3 minutes of tube placement.
- If there is some definite relief after applying the tube (>10%), then retain the tube in that position for 36 - 48 hours, its position must be well secured by an additional Band-aid-like tape. (It should neither be too tight to cause extra pressure nor too loose to move the tube from its place.)
- Displacement of the tube can decrease or even nullify the effect.
- Once removed, it must be reapplied for 8-10 hours every day, at the exact same location, until the problem entirely disappears.

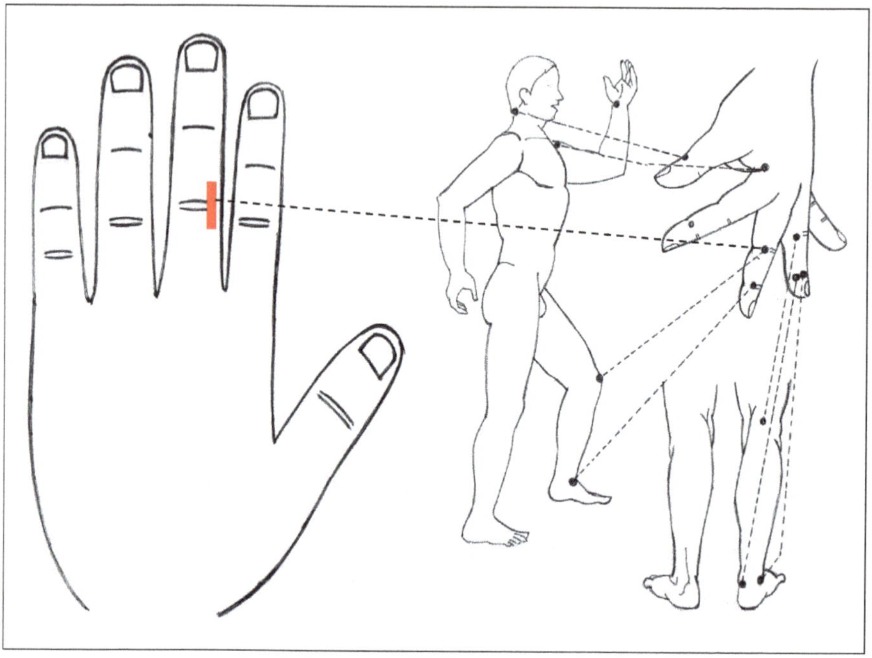

Fig 17.1: Tube Treatment for Left Chronic Knee Pain using Standard CR

Chronic Knee Pain - Ear Seeds

- Check the following ear points for tenderness with the help of a jimmy or point finder.
- These points are Knee CR, Kidney, Spleen, Muscle Relaxing point 1 (MR1)
- Ear seeds are applied at these points after cleaning the ear.
- These are retained for 2-3 weeks.

- The patient should be given instructions on care to be taken.
- This mode is mandatory in cases with osteoarthritis.

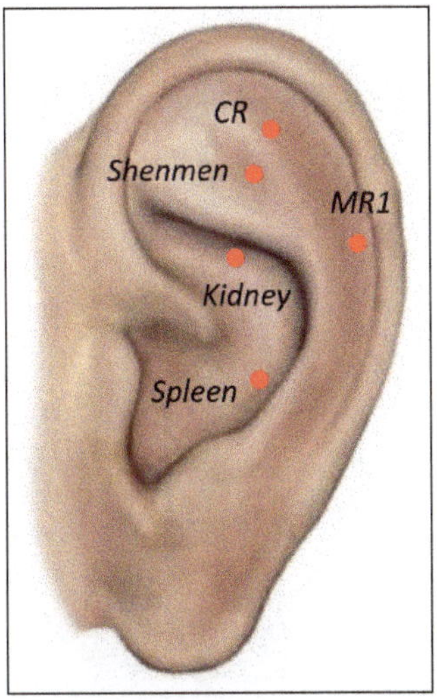

Fig 17.2: Ear Seeds Treatment for Left Chronic Knee Pain

Chronic Knee Pain - Bleeding

- Find out highly tender point on Standard CR with jimmy.
- Gently massage the point.
- Clean the area with alcohol (clinical spirit).
- Prick the point with a sterile blood-letting instrument and bleed 8 to 12 drops of blood with aseptic precautions.
- Apply a hollow plastic tube over the point that is bled. Follow tube protocol for further relief.

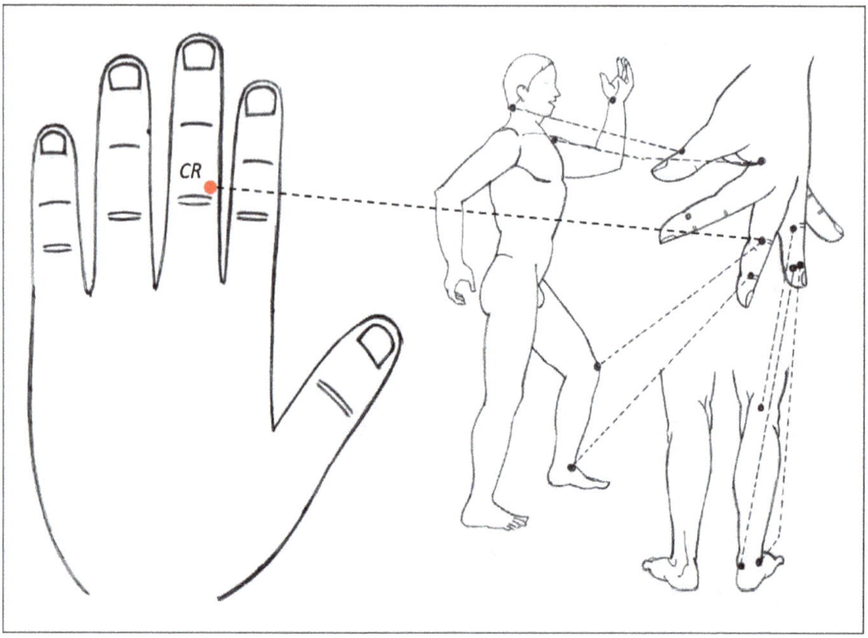

Fig 17.3: Bleeding Treatment for Left Chronic Knee Pain using Standard CR

Chronic Knee Pain - Acupoints

- Stimulate the following acupressure points by giving pressure with a jimmy on the same side hand as that of the pain.
- These points are ST36, ST45, GV4, UB23, K3, K7, LIV2, LIV8, UB11 and UB54.
- If the pain has not fully disappeared after stimulation with jimmy, then apply moong seeds on the same points with the germinating part (opening) touching the skin with an adhesive tape.

- On the first day, ask the patient to press these seeds 2 hourly for 30 times/minute. Remove them in the morning after pressing them again the same way.
- Subsequently, apply fresh seeds every night. Press them 30 times in one minute. Keep them overnight. Press them again after waking up in the morning and then remove the seeds.
- Continue for 2-20 days as required.
- After 20 days, give a break for 1week and then the seeds can be applied again.

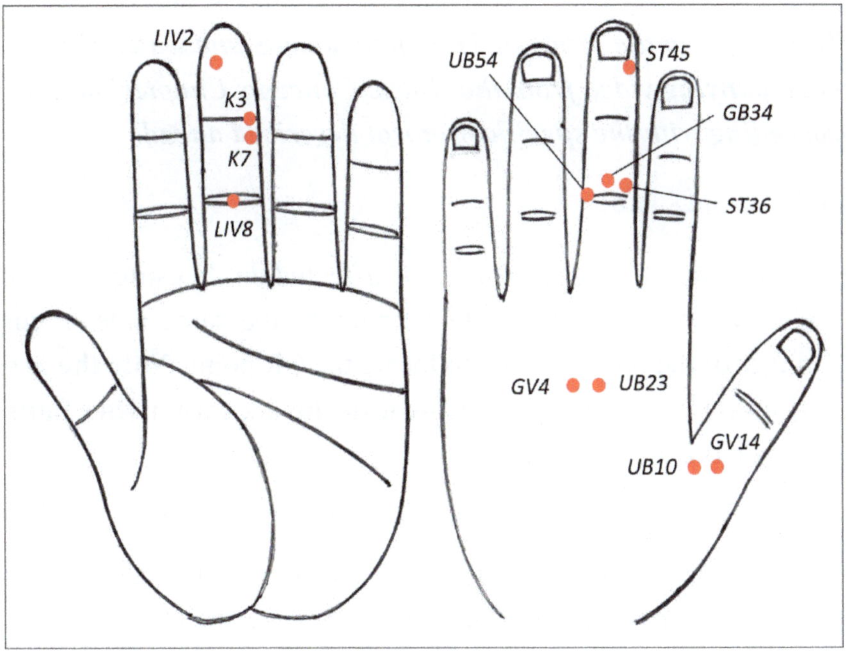

Fig 17.4: Acupoint Treatment for Left Chronic Knee Pain using Standard CR

18. Ankle Sprain

Introduction

A Patient comes with history of fall or twisting his ankle with

- Pain in ankle
- Swelling may be or may not be there
- Difficulty in walking

For this condition, tube application (along with bleeding if required) gave good results.

Please refer to the Mode of Treatment details and watch the accompanying video from the 'Basic Concepts Chapter' before proceeding with the specific protocol described ahead.

Ankle Sprain - Tube

- Roll Jimmy over the area of the affected ankle using Standard CR system along the middle finger of the same side or ring finger of the opposite side to locate the CR point. **Note the area of ankle CR carefully as shown in the accompanying figure as per the area of pain.**
- At times, there may be more than one painful point.
- Apply tube(s) with adhesive tape in the effective direction to cover each painful point (usually vertical) at the CR.
- Re-evaluate the pain and ask the patient to move the affected part after 2-3 minutes of tube placement.

- If there is some definite relief after applying the tube (>10%), then retain the tube in that position for 36 - 48 hours, its position must be well secured by an additional Band-aid-like tape. (It should neither be too tight to cause extra pressure nor too loose to move the tube from its place.)
- Displacement of the tube can decrease or even nullify the effect.
- Once removed, it must be reapplied for 8-10 hours every day, at the exact same location, until the problem completely disappears.

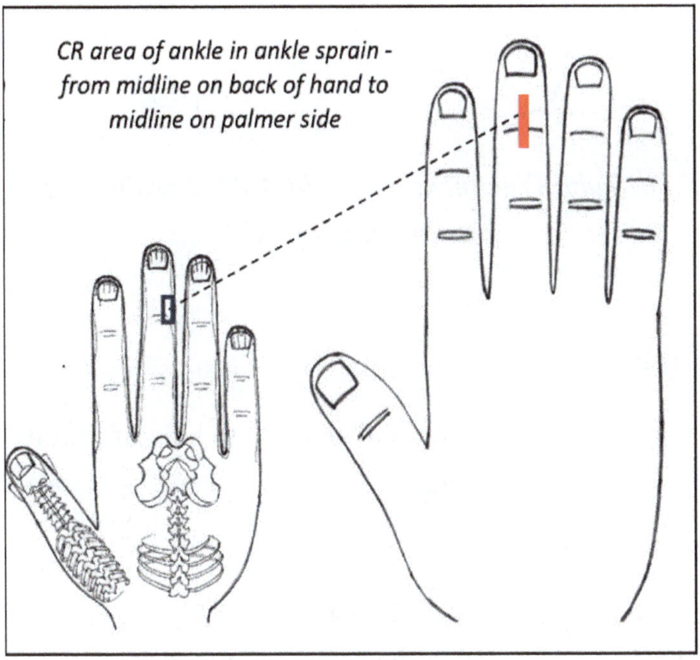

Fig 18.1a: Tube Treatment for Right Ankle Sprain on outer side using Standard CR

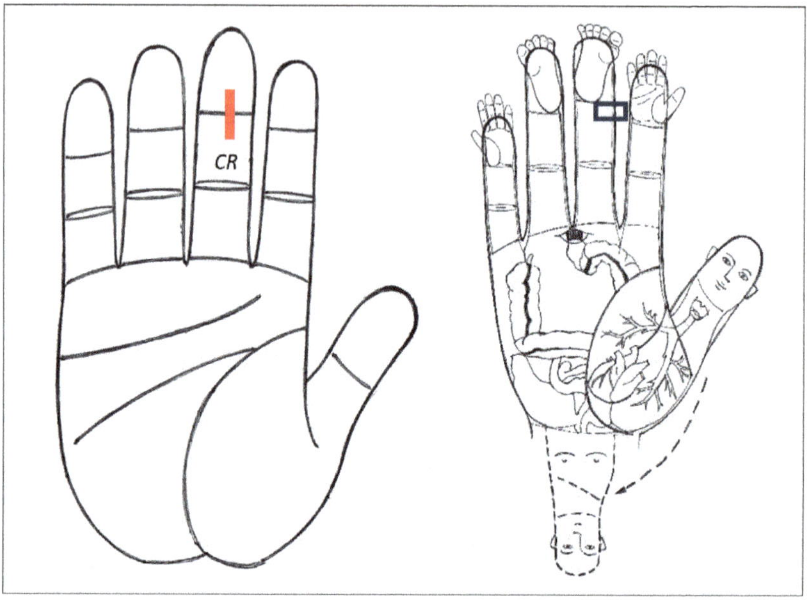

Fig 18.1b: Tube Treatment for Right Ankle Sprain on inner side using Standard CR

Ankle Sprain - Bleeding

- Find out the highly tender CR point with help of jimmy.
- Gently massage the point.
- Clean the area with alcohol (clinical spirit).
- Prick the point with a sterile blood-letting instrument and bleed 4 to 12 drops of blood with aseptic precautions.
- Apply a hollow plastic tube over the point that is bled. Follow tube protocol for further relief.

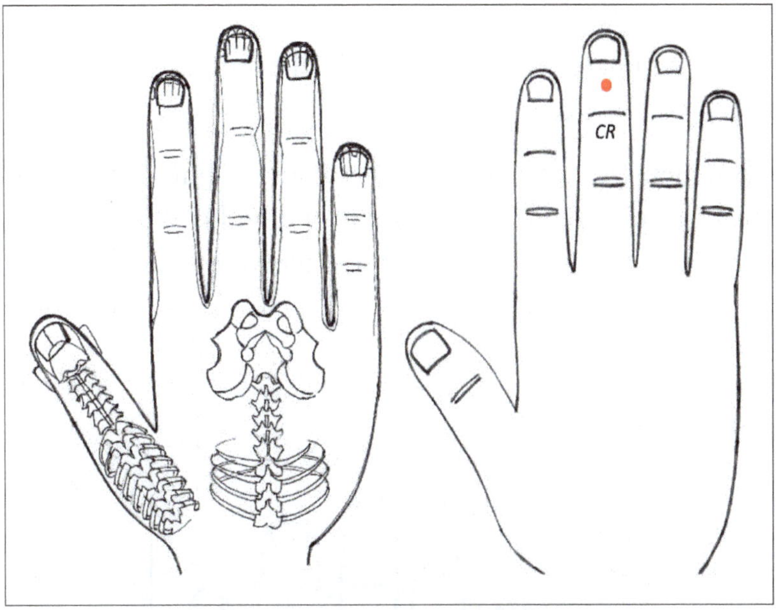

Fig 18.2: Bleeding Treatment for Right Ankle Sprain using Standard CR

Ankle Sprain - Acupoints

- Stimulate the following points by giving pressure with jimmy on the points - GB34 and Ah Shi point (most tender point) on ankle CR (in standard CR). Choose the same side hand as that of the pain.
- If the pain has not fully disappeared after stimulation with jimmy, then apply moong seeds on the same points with the germinating part (opening) touching the skin with an adhesive tape.

- On the first day, ask the patient to press these seeds 2 hourly for 30 times/minute. Remove them in the morning after pressing them again the same way.
- Subsequently, apply fresh seeds every night. Press them 30 times in one minute. Keep them overnight. Press them again after waking up in the morning and then remove the seeds.
- Continue for 2-20 days as required.
- After 20 days, give a break for 1week and then the seeds can be applied again.

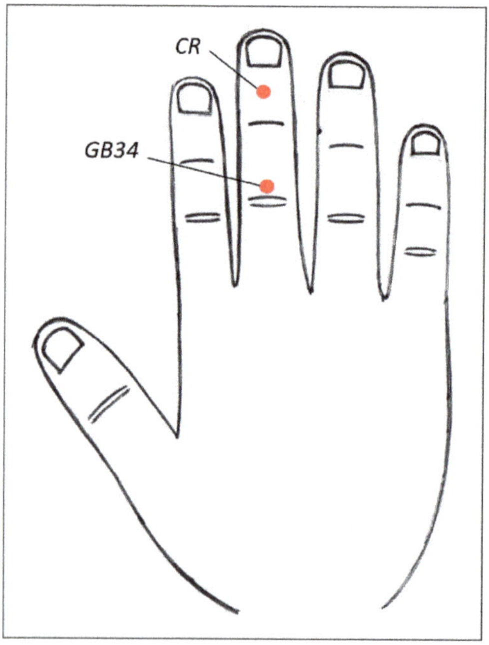

Fig 18.3: Acupoint Treatment for Right Ankle Sprain using Standard CR

19. Foot Pain

Introduction

Foot Pain is usually felt either on the sides or in the middle of the forefoot.

This can be initiated by wrong footwear, walking on uneven surfaces, fast/speedy walk or play or slight twist.

Proper history will reveal the cause, which should be addressed.

If the cause is not known, then advise proper padded footwear along with the protocol. This works well in most cases.

In this condition, tube application (along with bleeding if required) gave good results.

Please refer to the Mode of Treatment details and watch the accompanying video from the 'Basic Concepts Chapter' before proceeding for specific protocols described ahead.

Foot Pain - Tube

- Roll Jimmy over the area of affected Foot using Standard CR system along the middle finger of the same side or ring finger of the other hand.
- Identify the CR point and apply a hollow plastic tube with an adhesive tape in the effective direction (usually horizontal) at the CR point.

- Re-evaluate the pain and ask the patient to move the affected part after 2-3 minutes of tube placement.
- If there is some definite relief after applying the tube (>10%), then retain the tube in that position for 36 - 48 hours, its position must be well secured by an additional Band-aid-like tape. (It should neither be too tight to cause extra pressure nor too loose to move the tube from its place.)
- Movement of the tube can decrease or even nullify the effect.
- Once removed, it must be reapplied for 8-10 hours every day, at the exact same location, until the problem fully disappears.

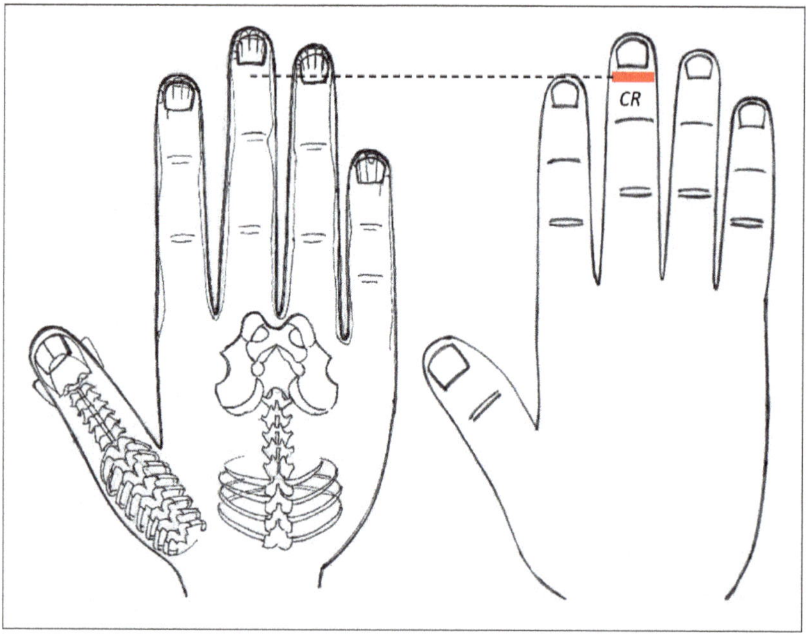

Fig 19.1: Tube Treatment for Right Foot Pain using Standard CR

Foot Pain - Ear Seeds

- Check the following ear points for tenderness with the help of jimmy or point finder.
- These points are Foot CR (behind the helix), Shenmen, Muscle Relaxing point 1 (MR1).
- Apply the ear seeds after cleaning the ear.
- These are to be retained for up to 2-3 weeks.
- Give instructions to patients on the care to be taken.

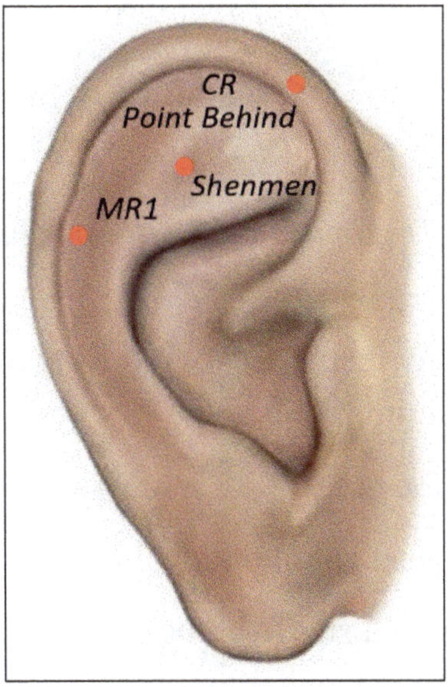

Fig 19.2: Ear Seeds Treatment for Right Foot Pain

Foot Pain - Bleeding

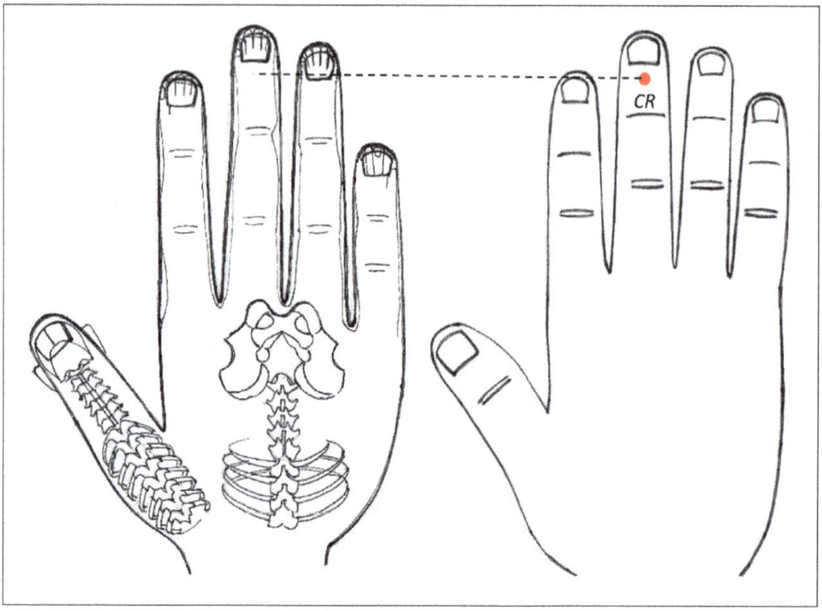

Fig 19.3: Bleeding Treatment for Right Foot Pain using Standard CR

- Find out the highly tender CR point using Standard CR system with the help of a jimmy.
- Gently massage the point.
- Clean the area with alcohol (clinical spirit).
- Prick the point with a sterile blood-letting instrument and bleed 4 to 10 drops of blood under aseptic precautions.
- Apply a hollow plastic tube over the point that is bled. Follow tube protocol for further relief.

Foot Pain - Acupoints

- Stimulate the following points by putting pressure with jimmy on the Byol meridians of the same side hand as that of the pain.
- These are CR, GB34, LIV2.
- If the pain has not fully disappeared after stimulation with jimmy, then apply moong seeds on the same points with the germinating part (opening) touching the skin with an adhesive tape.
- On the first day, ask the patient to press these seeds 2 hourly for 30 times/minute. Remove them in the morning after pressing them again the same way.
- Subsequently, apply fresh seeds every night. Press them 30 times in one minute. Keep them overnight. Press them again after waking up in the morning and then remove the seeds.
- Continue for 2-20 days as required.
- After 20 days, give a break for 1 week and then the seeds can be applied again.

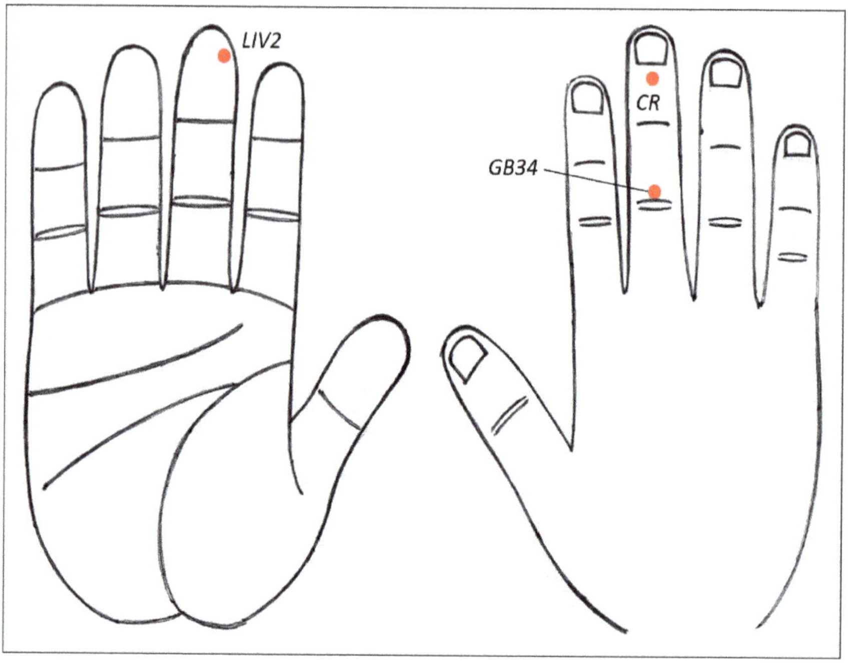

Fig 19.4: Acupoint Treatment for Right Foot Pain using Standard CR

20. TA (Achilles) Tendinitis

Introduction

The Pain at the back of the ankle or lower calf may signal a problem with the Achilles tendon (tendon of the calf muscles).

It can develop acutely stemming from inflammation of the tendon or tendon sheath (Tenosynovitis). Chronic cases occur because of painful scar tissue or imperfect healing of the injured tendon.

Acute condition heals faster. Chronic cases may take a longer time to heal. In this condition, tube application (along with bleeding if required) gave good results.

Please refer to the Mode of Treatment details and watch the accompanying video from the 'Basic Concepts Chapter' before proceeding for specific protocols described ahead.

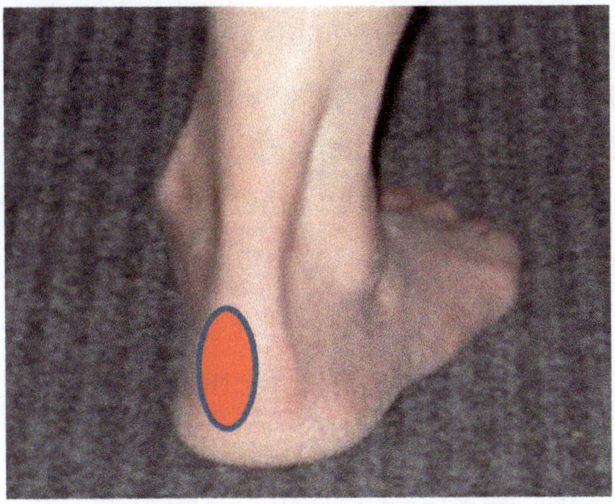

Fig 20: Achilles Tendinitis

TA Tendinitis - Tube

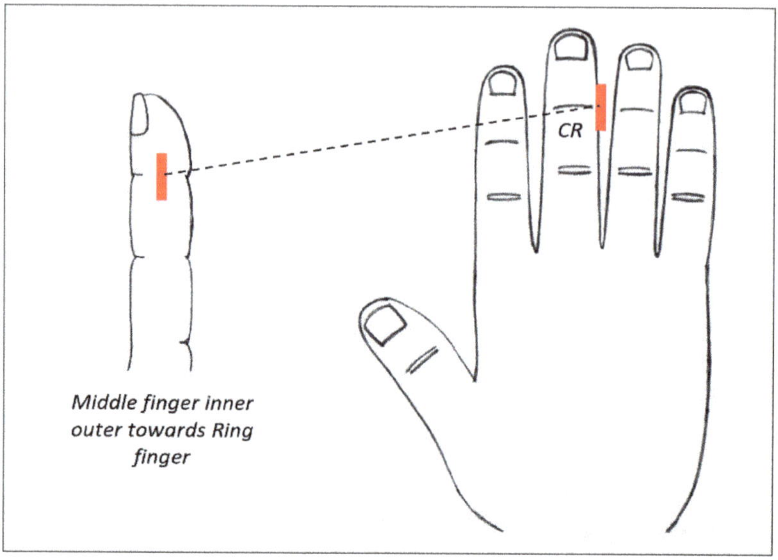

Fig 20.1: Tube Treatment for Right TA Tendinitis using Standard CR

- Roll Jimmy over the affected area using the Standard CR system. This is generally on the side of the finger. This can be found on the outer side of the middle finger of the same hand (as that of the side of pain) or the inner side of the ring finger of the opposite hand (as shown in the figure).
- Identify the CR point and apply a hollow plastic tube with an adhesive tape in the effective direction (usually Vertical) at CR point.
- Re-examine the pain and ask the patient to move the affected part after 2-3 minutes of tube placement.

- If there is some definite relief after applying the tube (>10%), then retain the tube in that position for 36 - 48 hours, its position must be well secured by an additional Band-aid-like tape. (It should neither be too tight to cause extra pressure nor too loose to move the tube from its place.)
- Movement of the tube can decrease or even nullify the effect.
- Once removed, it must be reapplied for 8-10 hours every day, at the exact same location, until the problem fully disappears.

TA Tendinitis - Bleeding

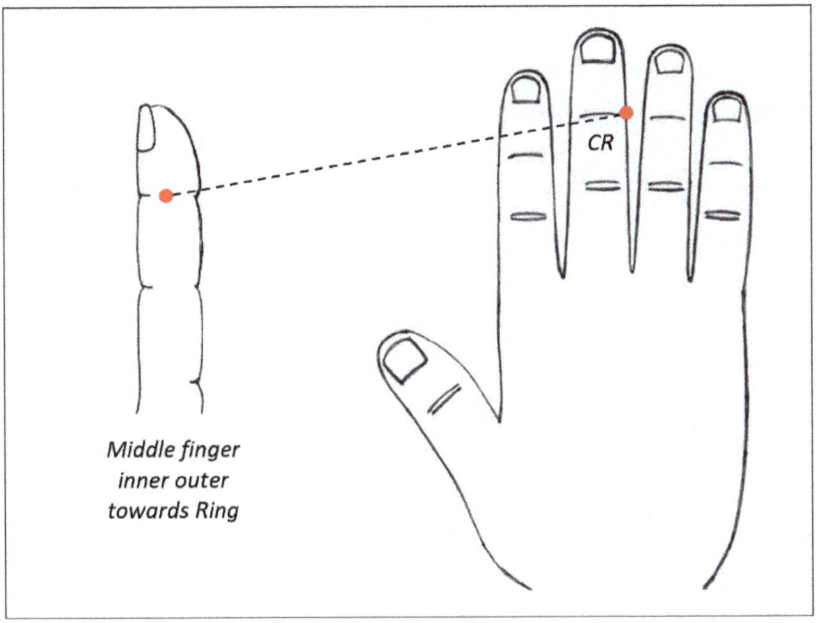

Fig 20.2: Treatment for Right TA Tendinitis using Standard CR on Left Ring Finger

- Identify the CR of the affected area using the Standard CR system. This is generally on the side of the finger. This can be found on the outer side of the middle finger of the same hand (as that of the side of pain) or the inner side of the ring finger of the opposite hand (as shown in the figure). Roll jimmy over it.
- Gently massage the point.
- Clean the area with alcohol (clinical spirit).
- Prick the point with a sterile blood-letting instrument and then bleed 2 to 10 drops of blood under aseptic precautions.
- Bleeding at this point usually gives significant instant relief.
- Apply a hollow plastic tube over the point that is bled. Follow tube protocol for further relief.

TA Tendinitis – Acupoints

- Stimulate the following points by creating pressure with jimmy on the Byol meridians of the same side hand as that of the pain.
- GB34, GB40, GB44 and CR (tender points on the area of correspondence)
- If the pain has not fully disappeared after stimulation with jimmy, then apply moong seeds on the same points with the germinating part (opening) touching the skin with an adhesive tape.

- On the first day, ask the patient to press these seeds 2 hourly for 30 times/minute. Remove them in the morning after pressing them again the same way.
- Subsequently, apply fresh seeds every night. Press them 30 times in one minute. Keep them overnight. Press them again after waking up in the morning and then remove the seeds.
- Continue for 2-20 days as required.
- After 20 days, give a break for 1 week and then the seeds can be applied again.

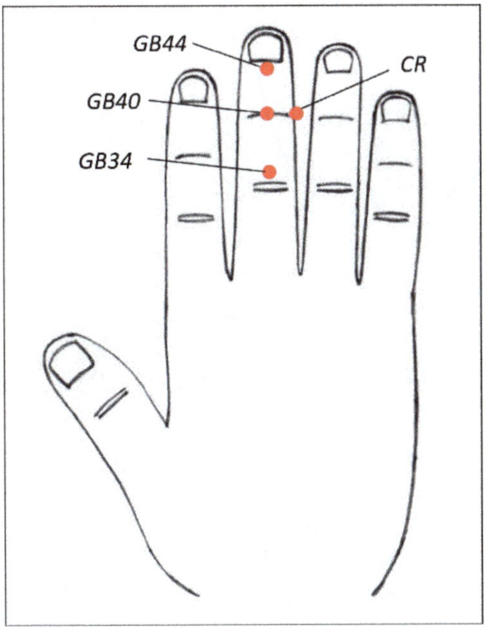

Fig 20.3: Acupoint Treatment for Right TA Tendinitis using Standard CR

TA Tendinitis – Wheat Seeds

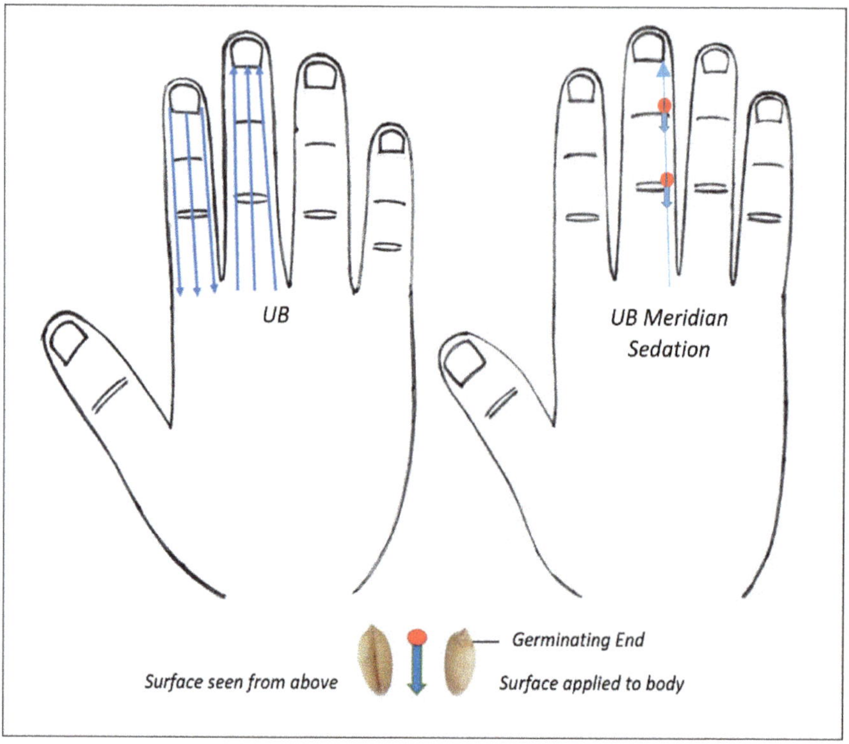

Fig 20.4: Wheat seed Treatment for Right TA Tendinitis on Right Hand

- Apply wheat seeds on the specified points such that the germinating end, where the red dot is shown in the figure, must be placed on the skin.
- After applying the wheat seed, ask the patient to wait for 20 minutes. Usually, there is some relief in symptoms during this

period. If there is no relief, then at least there should be no aggravation of the symptom. In case of aggravation, the wheat seeds should be removed immediately, and some other method should be tried.

- For the first 2 days, wheat seeds should be kept for 4-6 hours during the day. The patient is asked to confirm improvement before continuing this treatment.
- Every day use fresh wheat seeds.
- Continue for 2-20 days as required. The duration of the treatment should be tapered when more than 70% pain relief is experienced.
- Treatment should be discontinued once complete relief is obtained.

21. Heel Pain

Introduction

Patient complains of pain in the heel or around it and is unable to keep the heel on the ground, especially in the morning after waking up or after sitting for long time. Eventually, it may also be painful while walking.

This usually occurs due to plantar fasciitis - a frequent problem triggered by strain or micro injury to the fascia on the inner side of the foot, which helps in maintaining the arch of the foot.

This condition can be initiated by prolonged standing, inappropriate footwear, exercising on a hard surface. Address the above-mentioned causes appropriately to promote recovery. Also ensure that the Vitamin D status is good.

This protocol can give quick relief in most cases. In a few cases which did not respond to the EaseLife protocol methods, direct needling at the acupuncture points and the Ah Shi point (tender point) is beneficial.

For this condition, tube application (along with bleeding if required) was more effectivel.

Please refer to the Mode of Treatment details and watch the accompanying video from the 'Basic Concepts Chapter' before proceeding for specific protocols described ahead.

Heel Pain - Tube

- Roll jimmy on the area of affected heel in Standard CR system along the middle finger of the same side (as that of pain) or the ring finger of the opposite side.
- Apply a hollow plastic tube with adhesive tape in the effective direction (usually vertical) at the CR point.
- If there is some definite relief after applying the tube (>10%), then retain the tube in that position for 36 - 48 hours,
- If the relief is not substantial, then check for tenderness on the dorsal side (back side of the finger) just opposite the first tender point and apply one tube here also, simultaneously.
- Ask the patient if he has better relief with two tubes. If relief is better, then retain both the tubes in the same position for 36- 48 hours.
- Ensure that the tube position is well secured. Moving the tube from its place can decrease or even nullify the effect. If required, secure the tube using an additional adhesive non-toxic tape like Band-Aid. (It should neither be too tight to cause extra pressure nor loose so that the tube can move from its place.)
- If there is no significant relief of pain, then proceed for bleeding before application of the tube.
- Once the tube is removed it must be reapplied for 8-10 hours every day, at the same location, until the problem completely disappears.

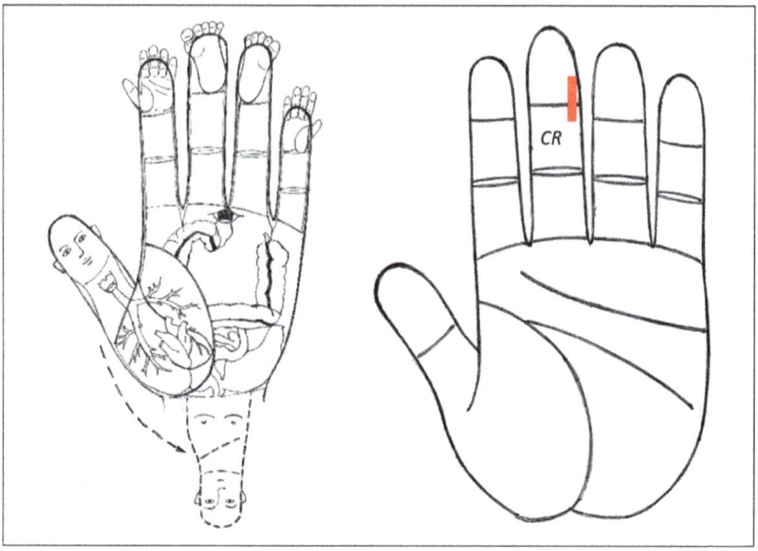

Fig 21.1a: Tube Treatment for Left heel pain using Standard CR

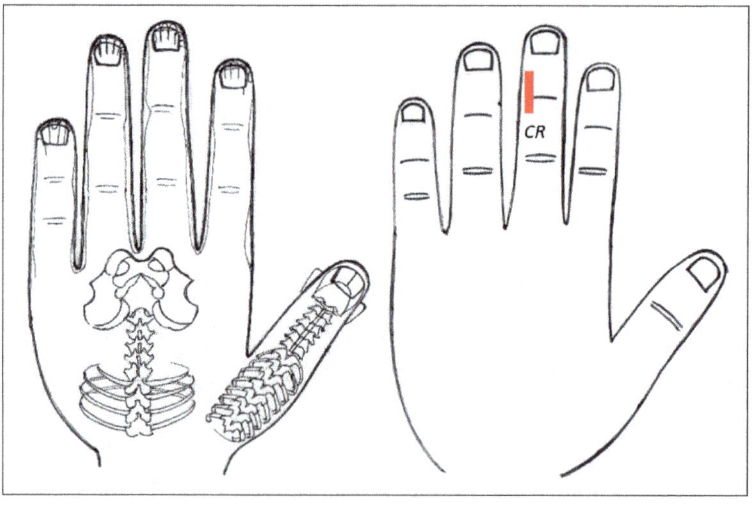

Fig 21.1b: Additional Tube Treatment for Left heel pain using Standard CR

Heel Pain - Bleeding

- Find out the highly tender CR point with help of jimmy.
- Gently massage the point.
- Clean the area with alcohol (clinical spirit).
- Prick the point with a sterile blood-letting instrument and then bleed 6 to 10 drops of blood under aseptic precautions.
- Apply a hollow plastic tube over the point that is bled. Follow tube protocol for further relief.

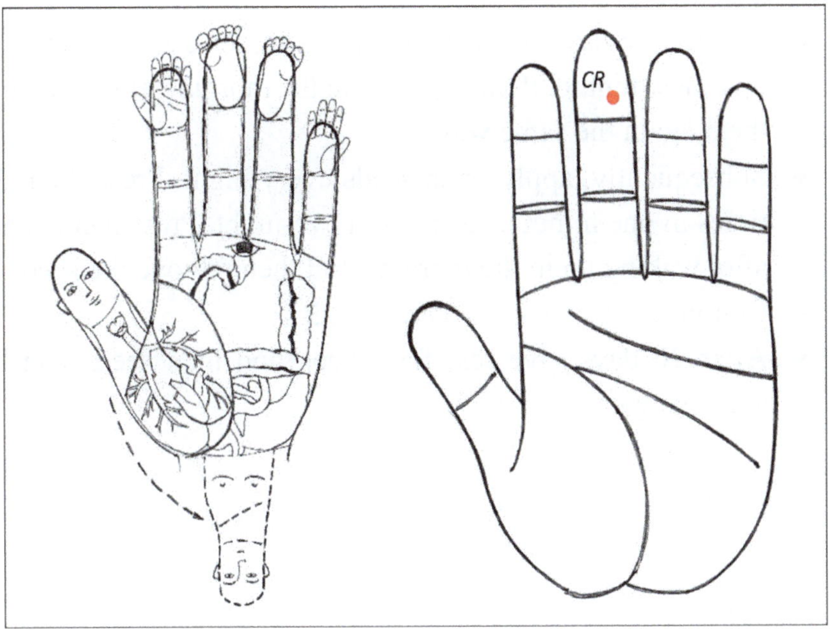

Fig 21.2: Bleeding Treatment for Left heel Pain using Standard CR

Heel Pain - Acupoints

- Stimulate the following points by giving pressure with jimmy on the Byol meridians of the same side hand as that of the pain.
- Liv2, K3, GB34, GB40, GB44 and Ah Shi point (tender point on the area of correspondence)
- If the pain has not fully disappeared after stimulation with jimmy, then apply moong seeds on the same points with the germinating part (opening) touching the skin with an adhesive tape.
- On the first day, ask patient to press these seeds 2 hourly for 30 times/minute. Remove them in the morning after pressing them again the same way.
- Subsequently, apply fresh seeds every night. Press them 30 times in one minute. Keep them overnight. Press them again after waking up in the morning and then remove the seeds.
- Continue for 2-20 days as required.
- After 20 days give rest for 1week and then seeds can be applied again.

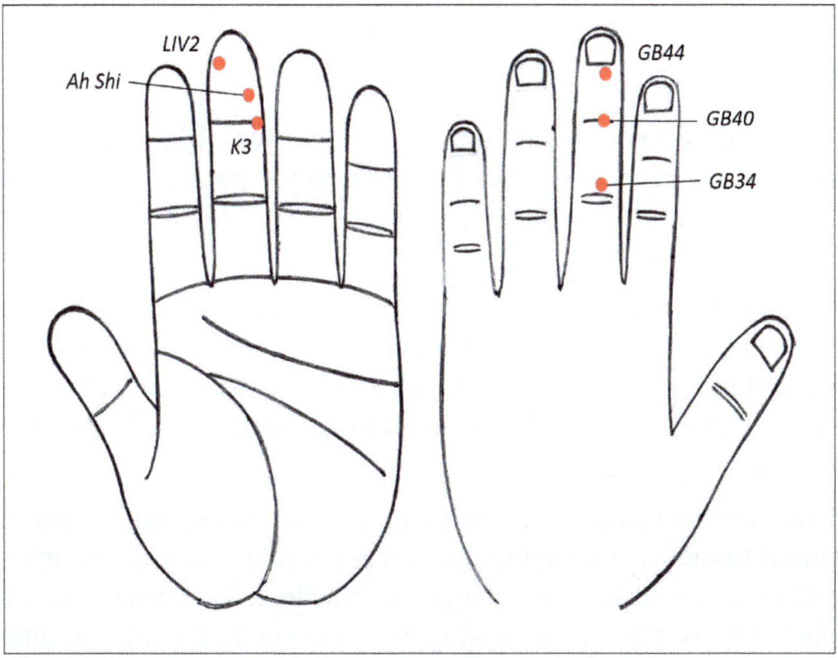

Fig 21.3: Acupoint Treatment for Left Heel Pain using Standard CR

22. Post Injury Pain Anywhere

Introduction

This condition occurs commonly in day-to-day life. Whenever a part of the body such as head / extremities / back etc. is hit with force, blunt injury results. This causes pain and swelling, which tends to increase with time.

The extent of injury to the tissue depends upon the magnitude of the striking force. The mechanical energy which remains in the injured tissues causes more damage and at the same time blocks the body's healing process. As a result, many a times, the misery of the patient increases the next day.

In this protocol, we drain the extra energy causing pain from the injured tissue by massaging the corresponding area with Jimmy or removing the locked-up energy by bleeding the correspondence point. Afterwards, the remaining extra damaging energy is drained through a plastic tube applied over the correspondence point. This has given significant relief in trauma cases.

Besides, applying ice to the local injured area which everyone knows reduces inflammation significantly. Ear seeds on the CR point, Shenmen (as anti-inflammatory point) can help further. The details of these modes are explained below.

For this condition, bleeding followed by tube application gave good results.

Please refer to the Mode of Treatment details and watch the accompanying video from the 'Basic Concepts Chapter' before proceeding for specific protocols described ahead.

Post Injury Pain on Right Hand - Tube

- Roll Jimmy over the area of injury on the palm using Standard CR or Insect CR system (preferably on the same side of the body where the problem exists).
- Apply a hollow plastic tube with adhesive tape in the effective direction at the CR point.
- Ask the patient to move the affected part and assess the pain after 2-3 minutes.
- If there is some definite relief after applying the tube (>10%), then retain the tube in that position for 36 - 48 hours, its position must be well secured by an additional Band-Aid like tape. (It should neither be too tight to cause extra pressure nor too loose to move the tube from its place.)
- Once removed it must be reapplied for 8-10 hours every day, at the same location, until the problem completely disappears.
- Normally, significant relief in pain is observed immediately and the remaining symptoms including residual pain resolve within 1-3 weeks of tube application.
- Moving the tube from its place can decrease or even nullify the effect.
- Normally, significant relief in pain is observed immediately and the remaining symptoms including residual pain resolve within 1-3 weeks of tube application.

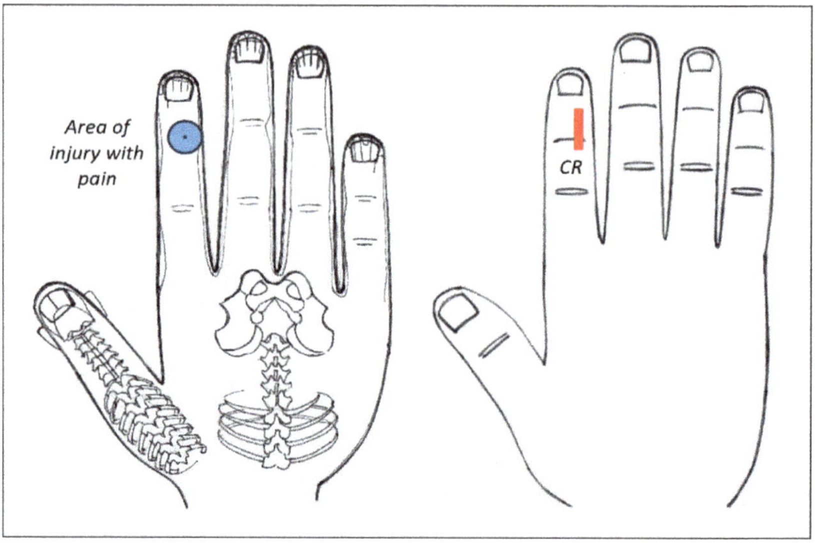

Fig 22.1a: Tube Treatment for Right Wrist Injury Pain using Standard CR

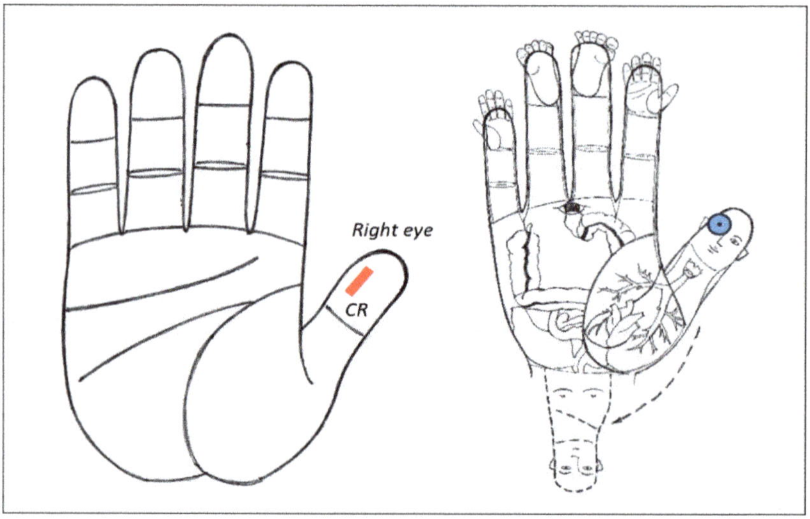

Fig 22.1b: Tube Treatment for Right Eye Injury Pain using Standard CR

Post Injury Pain on Right Hand - Bleeding

- In the cases of blunt injury, bleeding followed by Tube treatment helps get faster and better relief in post injury pain. (60-90% relief in 15 minutes)
- Find out with Jimmy the highly tender CR point.
- Gently massage the point.
- Clean the area with alcohol (clinical spirit).
- Prick the point with a sterile blood-letting instrument and then bleed 4 to 12 drops of blood with aseptic precautions.
- Apply a hollow plastic tube over the point that is bled. Follow tube protocol for further relief.

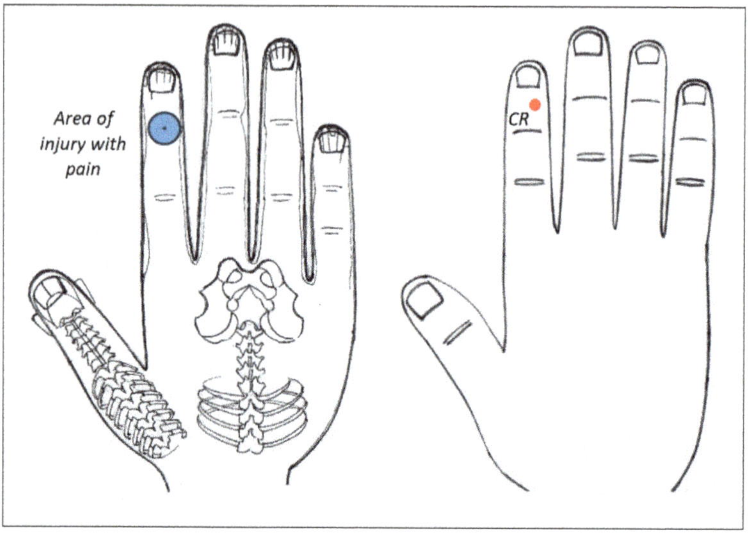

Fig 22.2a: Bleeding Treatment for Right Hand Injury Pain using Standard CR

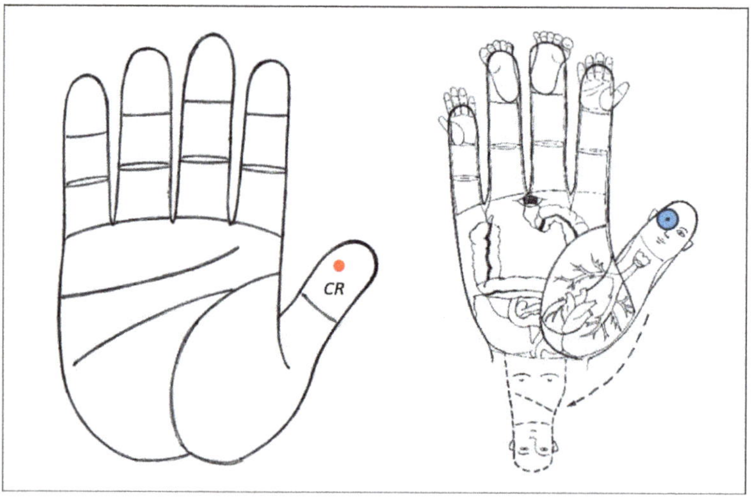

Fig 22.2b: Bleeding Treatment for Right Eye Injury Pain using Standard CR

23. One Sided Body Pain

Introduction

This condition appears frequently where the patient feels uneasiness or pain for a prolonged period in more than one part of the body on the same side (Left or Right). For example: Right side of the head, Right shoulder, Right arm, Right side of the chest, Right lumbar region, Right hip or Right knee - more than one of these issues are prevalent at a time. The other side is normal or without any complaints.

Here, the pain in different parts of the body on one side does not follow any meridian. There is excess energy which needs to be balanced with the other side. The transfer of energy is done with the help of pieces of plastic tube placed on the insect correspondence system.

We had a few patients who underwent various investigations which failed to give a diagnosis and hence no solution was offered. These patients improved completely after using this EaseLife protocol.

There is no such energy concept in modern medicine, so no specific diagnosis or treatment is provided.

Please refer to the Mode of Treatment details and watch the accompanying video from the 'Basic Concepts Chapter' before proceeding for specific protocols described ahead.

Body Imbalance - Tube

- Roll Jimmy over the area of the affected Insect CR i.e., on the side and on top of the finger.
- Insect CR of any finger (preferably index) can be used in this protocol (preferably on the same side of the body where the problem exists).
- Apply 3 pieces of tube with adhesive tape on the finger; 2 pieces of tube (in vertical position) besides the two interphalangeal joints and a smaller 3rd piece of tube on top of the finger in horizontal position as shown in the figure.
- Ask the patient to move the affected part and assess the pain after 2-3 minutes.
- If there is some definite relief after applying the tube (>10%), then retain the tube in that position for 36 – 48 hours, its position must be well secured by an additional Band-Aid like tape. (It should neither be too tight to cause extra pressure nor too loose to move the tube from its place).
- Moving the tube from its place can decrease or even nullify the effect.
- Once removed it must be reapplied for 8-10 hours every day, at the same location, until the problem completely disappears.
- Normally, significant relief in pain is observed immediately and the remaining symptoms including residual pain resolve within 1-3 weeks of tube application.

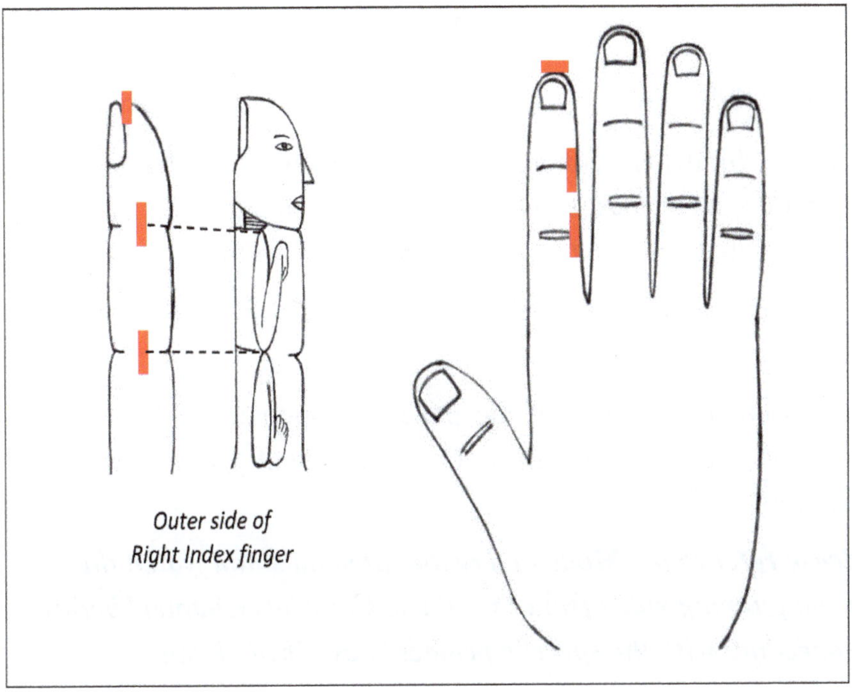

Fig 23.1: Tube Treatment for Right Side Body Imbalance using Insect CR

24. Allergic Rhinitis

Introduction

Allergic rhinitis is a condition where a person encounters symptoms such as excessive sneezing or running nose which may be associated with watery and itchy eyes and or throat.

Here is the protocol that helps most patients with allergic rhinitis in an easy way.

In this condition, 60% of the patients responded to LI meridian tonification and a few showed improvement with LI meridian sedation.

Please refer to the Mode of Treatment details and watch the accompanying video from the 'Basic Concepts Chapter' before proceeding with the specific protocol described ahead.

Allergic Rhinitis - Wheat seeds

- Allergic rhinitis can be mostly treated by tonifying the LI meridian. Occasionally, it needs to be sedated.
- Apply wheat seeds on the specified points such that the germinating end, where the red dot is shown in the figure, must be placed on the skin.
- Apply the seeds and wait for 20 minutes. The symptoms should start receding in 20 minutes. If so, continue to apply the seeds between 5:00 p.m. to 7:00 a.m. daily for a minimum of 3 to 4 days, and then you can apply it only while sleeping (7-8 hours).

- Do remember to use a new set of seeds for application the next day and discard used seeds.
- Stop doing this after complete recovery of the symptoms.
- If the symptoms worsen, reverse the direction of wheat grains, and observe for the next half an hour. Continue applying the seeds for the above-mentioned duration if this direction works.

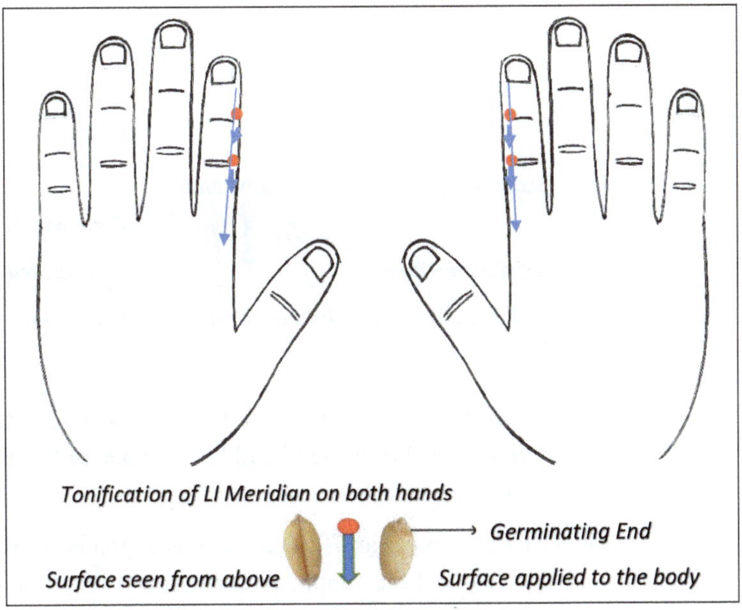

- *Fig 24.1a: Wheat Seed Treatment of Allergic Rhinitis*

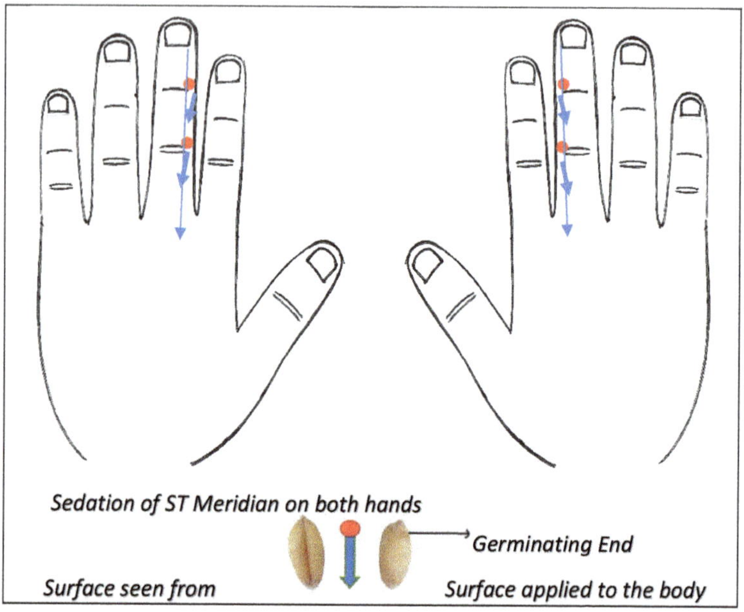

Fig 24.1b: Additional Wheat Seed Treatment of Allergic Rhinitis

- If both the above approaches do not work, then the stomach meridian can be sedated in addition to one of the above methods and tried.
- Usually, more than 70% recovery is appreciated over the first 4 days if wheat seed application has shown improvement on the first day.

25. Sinus Headache

Introduction

This is a condition where the patient complains of a headache on one side of the face above or below the eye for a few days.

This subsides with a painkiller for a short duration but can recur later.

Sometimes, it can occur on both sides.

It gets aggravated by bending down and has been observed to increase at a particular time of the day in most patients.

The patient may give a history of an occurrence of cold in the past few days (either due to allergy or infection).

Applying pressure over the sinus area and on the side of the base of the nose causes pain.

Please refer to the Mode of Treatment details and watch the accompanying video from the 'Basic Concepts Chapter' before proceeding to the specific protocols described ahead.

Sinus Headache - Bleeding

- Roll Jimmy over the area of the nose in insect CR of any finger.
- Mark the most painful point in that area of correspondence.
- Gently massage the point.
- Clean the area with alcohol (clinical spirit).
- Prick the point with a sterile lancet and bleed 8 to 12 drops of blood with aseptic precautions.
- Apply a hollow plastic tube over the point that is bled in a vertical direction (follow tube protocol) for further relief.
- Ask the patient to assess the headache after 5 minutes of tube application.
- If there is some definite relief, then retain the tube in that position for 36 - 48 hours. Its position must be well secured by adhesive bandages like Band-Aid tape.
- The same tube can be reapplied daily at the aforesaid point for 10 hours till the problem disappears completely.
- Rarely, the procedure of bleeding from nose CR of the other finger may be repeated on the second or third day if there is only partial relief.

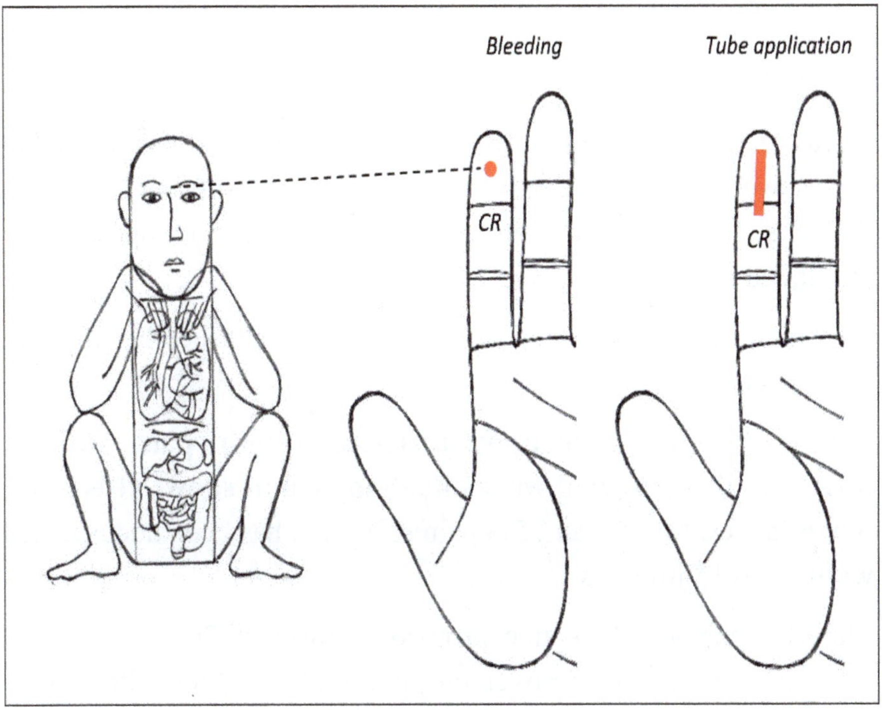

Fig 25.1: Bleeding followed by Tube Treatment for Sinus Headache using insect CR

26. Third molar (wisdom tooth) Pain

Introduction

Occasionally, the eruption of the third molar (wisdom tooth) can cause swelling of the gums around it and lead to substantial pain in the jaws, gums, and head and affecting activities like opening the mouth, eating, drinking, etc.

This may become severe at times even in the absence of infection in the tooth.

For this type of eruption-associated tooth pain without infection, this protocol works like magic and shows effect in a few minutes. More than 75% pain reduction has been documented within 5 to 15 minutes.

Majority responded to tube protocol. However, 20% of patients who showed <50% improvement, required bleeding followed by tube protocol.

Please refer to the Mode of Treatment details and watch the accompanying video from the 'Basic Concepts Chapter' before proceeding with the specific protocol described ahead.

Wisdom tooth Pain - Tube

- For wisdom tooth pain, we use the animal correspondence system of Sujok. For this method, any finger can be used.
- Note the location of the correspondence of the different molars - upper and lower, right and left in the figure given below.
- With the help of Jimmy, identify the most tender point on a particular tooth correspondence around the nail. Mark it with a pen.
- Apply the plastic tube on it in a slanting/curved way to cover the point near the nail corner firmly with an adhesive tape.
- If there is some relief after 5 minutes, then retain the tube in the same position for 36 - 48 hours with the help of an additional tape like Band-Aid over it to hold it in the same position.
- Displacement of the tube can decrease or even nullify the effect.
- Typically, the pain disappears in 48 hours but in case it persists, then reapply the tube every day for 8 to 10 hours in the same location until it disappears completely.

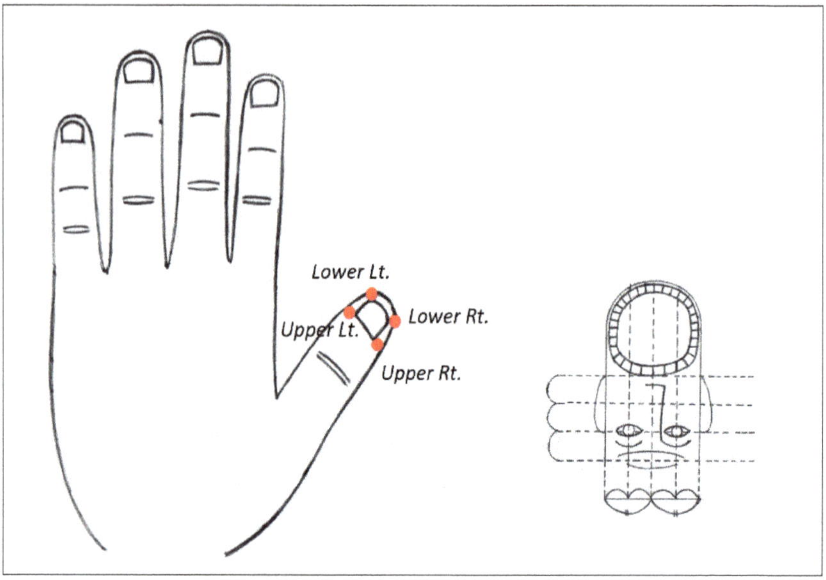

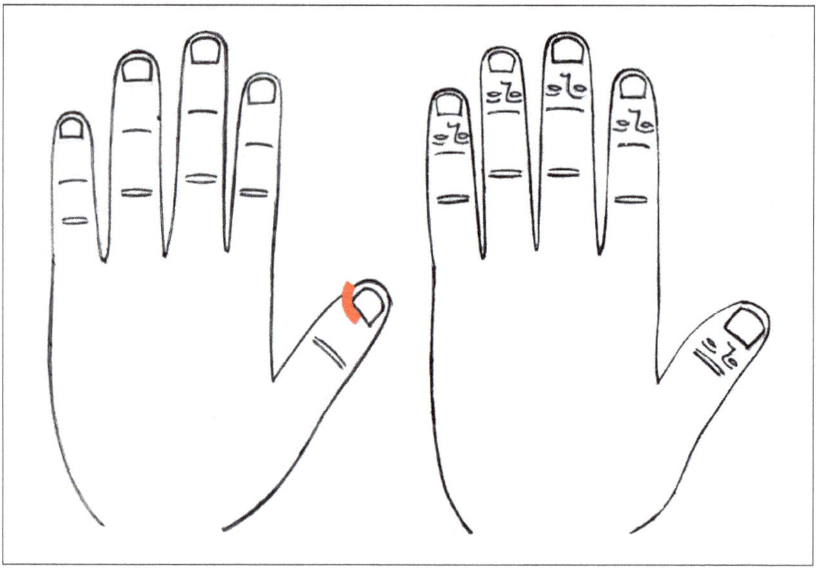

Fig 26.1 Tube Treatment for Left Upper Wisdom tooth Pain on Animal CR

27. Vertigo

Introduction

Vertigo is an abnormal sensation of motion where the person feels as if the world around him is spinning.

It can be of two types- central (brain-related) and peripheral (balancing apparatus or nerve-related).

Benign paroxysmal positional vertigo (BPPV) which is a peripheral cause of vertigo is the commonest variety we see.

This protocol is only for Benign paroxysmal positional vertigo (BPPV).

This is due to disturbance in the vestibular apparatus in the inner ear which is responsible for creating a sense of balance in the body.

Around 40% of the patients responded to tube protocol and 25% responded to ear seed application.

Please refer to the Mode of Treatment details and watch the accompanying video from the 'Basic Concepts Chapter' before proceeding with the specific protocol described ahead.

Vertigo - Tube

- Roll Jimmy over areas of both ears CR in insect CR of any finger, preferably the index finger. The pressure usually gives a variable amount of pain.

- Apply two plastic hollow tubes in a vertical direction on both ear CR areas of the same finger and assess vertigo after 15 minutes. If there is definite relief (usually more than 50%), retain the tubes for 36 to 48 hours.
- The tubes must be well secured by a band-aid like tape. It should neither be too tight to cause too much pressure nor too loose to cause displacement.
- Moving the tube from its place can decrease or even nullify the effect.
- The tubes should be reapplied for 8 to 10 hours every day at the same point until vertigo resolves.

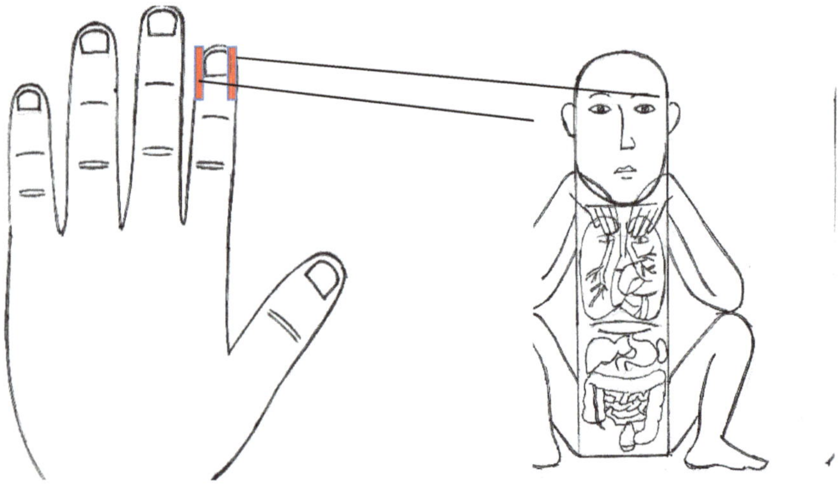

Fig 27.1: Tube Treatment of Acute Vertigo (BPPV) using Insect CR

Vertigo - Ear Seeds

- Check the following ear point for tenderness with the help of Jimmy or point finder.
- Ear seeds are placed on one or both ears, whichever has a tender 'inner ear' point after cleaning the ear.
- If there is relief, these ear seeds are retained for 2 to 3 weeks.
- The patient should be given instructions on care to be taken.

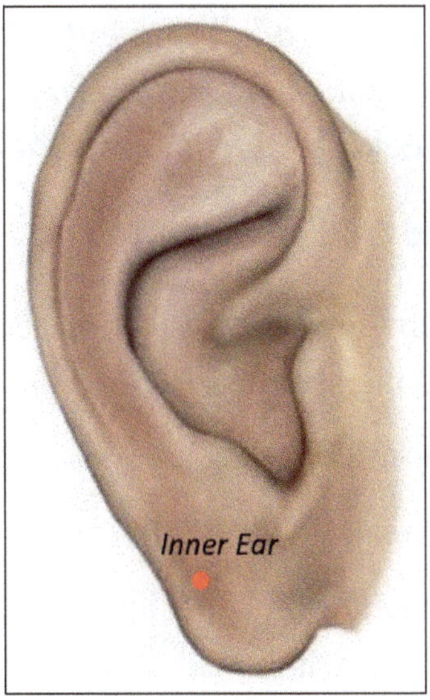

Fig 27.2: Ear Seed Treatment of Acute Vertigo (BPPV)

28. Recurrent Cough and Cold

Introduction

This protocol is applicable for repeated episodes of bronchitis, asthmatic bronchitis, and asthma particularly in children which can be well controlled by stimulating the subsequent acupressure points that take care of the lung and its supporting structures.

90% of the children who followed the protocol properly, responded extremely well to this treatment.

Please refer to the Mode of Treatment details and watch the accompanying video from the 'Basic Concepts Chapter' before proceeding to the specific protocol described ahead.

Recurrent Cough and Cold - Acupoints

- Stimulate the following points given in the figure with healthy green gram or moong seeds.

  LI4, LI11, LU5, LU9, SP10, K3, CV17, GV14, UB13

- It is better to first mark these points with a pen.
- The author recommends mehendi application on these points for 20 minutes to an hour which will leave an orange stain for about 4-5 days which will make identification of these points easy for seed application.
- Place fresh green gram or moong with its opening touching the skin on each point with adhesive tape.

- Press each moong, with tolerable pressure, for about 30 times a minute.
- Press the remaining points in the same manner.
- Keep the seeds for 6 to 8 hours (preferably overnight), and after 8 hours, press each seed again 30 times a minute and then remove and throw the seeds.
- Apply new moong seeds on the points the next day.
- If the problem is severe, apply seeds on both hands for one or two days followed by alternate hands on the succeeding days.
- Generally, the results are seen from the first day of placement of seeds.
- The duration of this therapy varies from person to person. It can last anywhere between 6 weeks to 3 months after which children will stop getting cough attacks. Even if the child gets a subsequent cough attack, it will be controlled by this seed therapy easily.
- In the last 15 years of my practice, we did not put any child (between 1 to 12 years) on an inhaler for asthma or asthma-like cough.
- **Note:** Although this method is tedious and children may refuse to press the seeds on tender points initially, the results are promising. If the child throws away the seeds after pressing, reapply and press them 3 times a day for the first 2-3 days. The

child starts showing improvement from the second day of treatment and they soon start cooperating with this therapy.

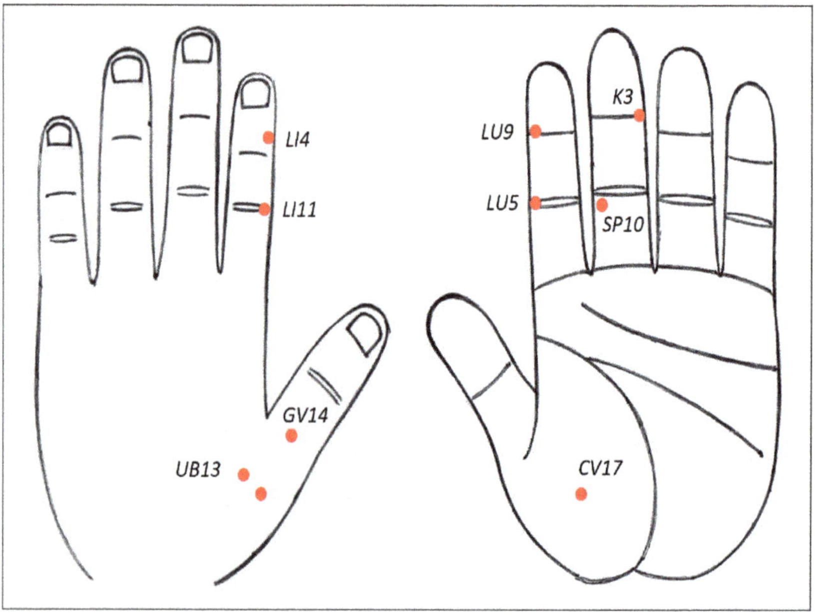

Fig 28.1: Acupoint Treatment for Recurrent Cough and Cold on Byol Meridian

Annexure 1 - Clinical Data

Sr No	Condition	# of Patients	Recovery Period				# of Patients Cured
			Immediate	< 1 Week	< 2 Weeks	> 2 Weeks	
1	Acute neck sprain	50	25	16	5	0	46
2	Acute neck pain	50	6	20	16	2	44
3	Acute backache	60	15	13	12	14	54
4	Acute shoulder pain	60	10	16	17	5	48
5	Frozen shoulder	61	3	10	24	19	56
6	Elbow tendinitis	63	14	16	26	4	60
7	Wrist & Thumb pain	28	7	0	16	2	25
8	Carpal tunnel syndrome	22	8	6	4	2	20
9	Acute UE pain along meridian	52	28	19	2	0	49
10	Trigger finger	18	0	3	6	5	14
11	Acute lower backache	40	8	7	22	0	37
12	Acute lumbar pain	40	13	10	12	1	36
13	Chronic backache	72	8	5	17	35	65
14	Tailbone pain	11	3	5	2	0	10
15	Sciatica	51	9	10	15	12	46
16	Acute knee pain	39	5	6	11	8	30
17	Chronic knee pain	72	6	7	17	26	56
18	Ankle sprain	52	8	33	2	3	46
19	Foot pain	21	6	6	3	4	19
20	Achilles tendinitis	24	1	7	4	8	20
21	Heel pain	50	0	17	21	7	45
22	Post blunt injury pain	25	2	15	3	3	23
23	Body imbalance	33	3	11	10	6	30
24	Sinus headache	24	6	14	0	0	20
25	Allergic rhinitis	20	0	12	3	0	15
26	Wisdom tooth pain	18	8	9	0	0	17
27	Vertigo	12	4	3	0	0	7
28	Recurrent cough and cold	44	0	0	0	41	41

www.ingramcontent.com/pod-product-compliance
Ingram Content Group UK Ltd.
Pitfield, Milton Keynes, MK11 3LW, UK
UKHW021337190726
13845UKWH00027B/600

9 789334 076905